Essential Oils Collection:

Learn Essential Oils Blends For Multiple Use, Make Soap and Natural Fresh Deo

Table of Content :

Book 1:

Book 2:

Book 3:

Book 4:

Book 5:

Book 6:

Book 7:

Book 8:

ESSENTIAL OILS FOR WEIGHT LOSS:

LOSE WEIGHT, BURN FAT AND BE FULL OF ENERGY

ROSIE GRAHAM

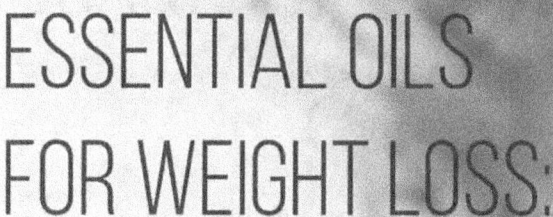

Essential Oils for Weight Loss:

Lose Weight, Burn Fat and Be Full of Energy

Introduction

Essential oils have been a recent trend among people whether celebrities or not who are interested in losing some weight. Weight loss is good whether for health purpose or the sake of good looks.

Essential oils are natural yet powerful. Also, they are easier to follow compared to diets that alter regular feeding style. The research on essential oils is ongoing with many exciting discoveries already made.Apart from the fact that essential oils are effective for weight loss, they are also useful in achieving balanced emotions, appetite control as well as a good scent for your body.

In this book, you'll find a short discussion about how essential oils work, why they work, some essential oils and how to use them as well as some essential oils recipes that you can make from the comfort of your home. That's a major advantage of essential oils the ease of preparation.

This book also mentions how you can work essential oils into your bracelet and necklace using ceramic diffuser beads to hold the scent of your essential oil all day.

I wish you success on your journey to weight loss using essential oils.

Chapter 1 – Why Essential Oils work

Different cultures from various parts of the world have known about the benefits essential oils have some of which are therapeutic and can heal. The abilities of the essential oil have been in full use for over 6000 years some to countries and empires like the Greeks, Chinese, Romans, Indians and so much more.

The essential oils are from various parts on a plant or tree. There are essential oils that they extract from the root, stem, bark, flowers and fruits. And for this reason, the essential oils in themselves will have different features that distinguish them from others.

A good example will be the essential oils that are known to have strong anti-inflammation properties, while others can be insecticidal or anti-microbial. In this light, there are also some essential oils that fat burning capabilities or help to curb cravings or unnecessary appetite.

How Essential Oils Work For Weight Loss

Your brain contains parts that are responsible for putting your body in the best physical shape and the right mental state, such that the when you stimulate these parts of the brain properly there are some have a general positive on you as an individual and this practice is known as *Aromatherapy*.

The human nose contains receptors that can perceive trillions of different kinds of smell, and they also have a crucial function of communicating to the amygdala and hippocampus in the brain, which are essential places where you keep memories and information.

Now for every inhalation of essential oils, study suggests that the amygdala and hippocampus are greatly affected such that they, in turn, influence our emotional and physical states almost instantly and directly, some of which are our motivation, mood, stress and sleep.

Even though presently there is no substitute for a healthy diet and regular exercising to help with weight loss, essential oils can go a long way to help with your weight loss target.

So eventually whether or not you fight a constant battle with cravings, low moods, slow metabolism, fatigue and emotional eating, essential oils can be that missing ingredient you need to achieve your weight loss target.

Chapter 2 – How to Use Oil Essentials for Weight Loss

Research by the Smell and Taste Treatment along with the Research Institute of Chicago resonated around the fact that continually inhaling culinary smell throughout the day (3-6 times)can go a long way in suppressing the desire to eat or taste anything especially when hungry.

Furthermore, the research advised that you should continue to change the essential oil you use across the day as this will help you to avoid the problem of familiarity with the essential oil, this will also bring a higher degree of efficiency.Here are some essential oils that can help you lose weight

Types of Essential Oil and How to Use Them

Cinnamon Essential Oil

It won't be strange to find that most people with diabetes use this oil.A study done in 2013 indicated that cinnamon "has anti-parasitic, anti-oxidant, anti-microbial and free radical scavenging properties".And also that it tends to reduce serum cholesterol and blood glucose.

The study also indicates that cinnamon oil has excellent abilities in stabilizing blood glucose level and Glucose Tolerance Factor (GTF) in the body, this is essential because blood sugar levels could also lead to over-eating, lower energy levels, weight gain, sugar craving and even irritability.By adding cinnamon oil to food, it can help in slowing down the rate by which glucose flows into your bloodstream, and this will help you in achieving your weight goals in the long run.

Cinnamon leaf oil contains eugenol, and this alters the neurosensory perceptions and also affect the way we taste and smell food, and this will help to reduce food craving and also stop overeating.

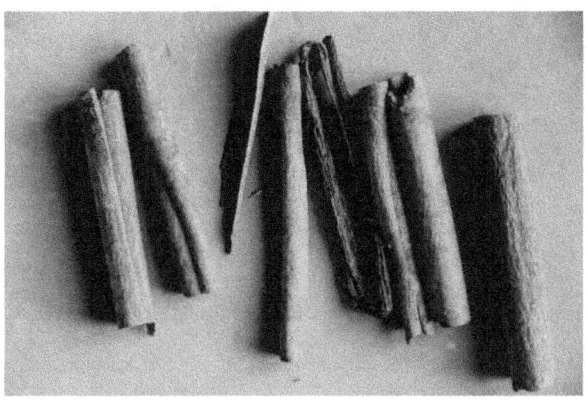

Using Cinnamon Essential Oil for Weight Loss:

- By drinking it: the FDA recommends that the cinnamon oil is safe to take directly internally, but it is advisable that you buy therapeutic-grade cinnamon essential oil.Therapeutic-grade cinnamon essential oil is 100% pure and toxin and addictive free.

Therapeutic-grade cinnamon essential oil is unfiltered and undiluted. You can also add 1 to 2 drops of cinnamon oil into warm water (about a teacup) with a little touch of honey (raw honey would work fine and better) to help in the fat loss.If you do this daily, it helps in reducing cravings. To curb late night food craving, it is advisable that have it before a meal or when the craving for food surfaces. You can also add cinnamon oil to your oats, baking or smoothies.

- Inhale directly: to prevent overeating before a meal or whenever a sudden carving sets in, you can inhale some cinnamon oil straight out of the bottle. As you do this regularly, it could go a great deal in improving your mood and make you fuller. It is advisable for emotional eaters.

- Apply topically: mix one to two drops of cinnamon oil with either of coconut oil or jojoba oil. After you do this, apply by rubbing it on your chest and wrist.

- Diffuse: put drops of cinnamon oil into your diffuser as this will not only give the house a great smell but will also help to stimulate a good mood.

Lemon Essential Oil

Lemon essential oils are known to be extracted from the lemon skin and containing the compound limonene, which makes lemon oil a characteristic fat dissolver.A recent report recommended that when joined with grapefruit oil, lemon oil supported lipolysis (separating of body fats) making it a "suppression in body weight gain."

Lemon oil additionally detoxifies and take out poisons in the body that can be stored in the fat cells, slow down parasites in the intestines, and improve digestion.

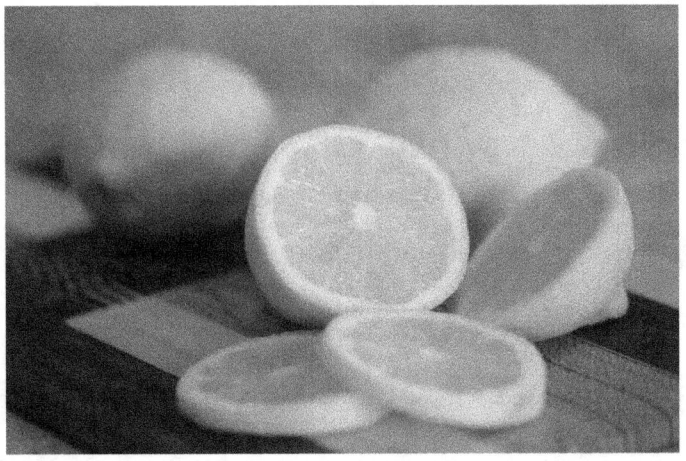

<u>Using Lemon Essential Oil for Weight Loss</u>

- Mix 2 drops of lemon oil to a glass of water in the morning and drink, this will help in detoxifying. It also supports digestion.

- Inhale the lemon directly from the bottle or soak cotton balls into the container and inhale directly from the cotton balls, this will curb cravings for food and decrease overeating.

- Blend the lemon oil with oils like coconut oil (carrier oil) and massage the mixture into areas that contain cellulite build-up.

Bergamot Essential Oil

Nervousness, gloom and low moods are frequently the major causes with regards to emotional eatingGiving in to your cravings may help light up your state of mind in the short term span yet over the long haul it just prompts sentiments of blame and low esteem, particularly when you heap on the pounds.

An ongoing 2015 investigation inferred that simply breathing in bergamot oil for 15 minutes can help your state of mind as well as decrease cortisol (a pressure hormone), that has a negative impact on fat loss.

In a recent report, 237 members with hyperlipemia (elevated amounts of fat in the blood) were given a fresh extract of bergamot orally for 30 days, and the investigation demonstrated that they could diminish blood cholesterol levels and altogether help in the reduction of blood glucose.

Bergamot contains polyphenols (a similar compound found in green tea), and it can push the body to dissolve fat and sugar normally. The sweet citrus aroma of bergamot oil gives you a high sense of feel, causing you to unwind and also smother cravings and control emotional eating.

Bergamot also has an enormous amount of limonene (additionally found in grapefruit oil and lemon oil), bergamot oil can burn fat. As indicated by University Health News, "D-limonene goes about as a gentle appetite suppressant and counteracts weight gain."

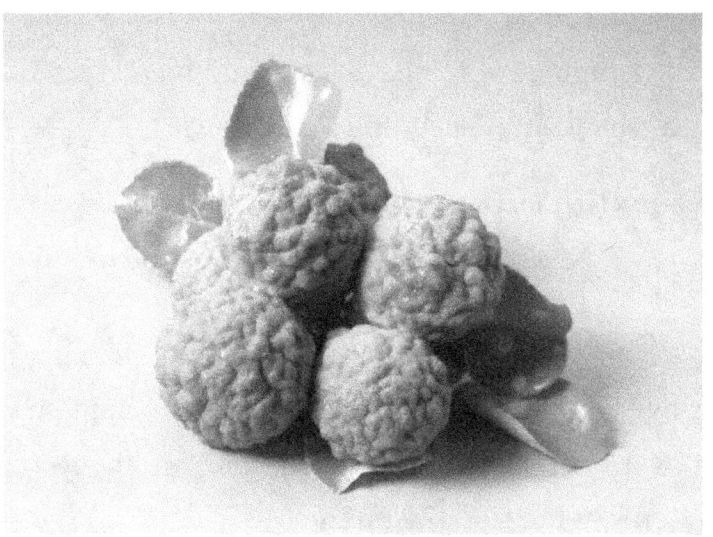

Using Bergamot Essential Oil for Weight Loss

- Inhale the oil directly or use a cotton ball soaked in oil, this scent of limonene will help to suppress cravings which in turn helps you to lose weight.

- Add this essential oil to your shower and cover the drain, inhale the scent to get the maximum benefits which keep you refreshed and in the right mind to lose weight.

Frankincense Essential Oil

Frankincense oil is gotten from the native of a tree local to Somalia, in Africa, and is fantastic for calming uneasiness and low inclinations that can trigger the need to eat more to food to feel satisfied.

Wealthy in sub-atomic structures called sesquiterpenes, that can cross the blood-cerebrum boundary, frankincense oil can ease the negative impacts of both uneasiness and misery.

Frankincense oil can encourage digestion by accelerating the flow rate of bile and gastric juices which in turn influences the metabolic rate and helps weight reductionIt can likewise stimulate peristaltic movement which enables food to move quickly through the digestive organs, improving digestion.

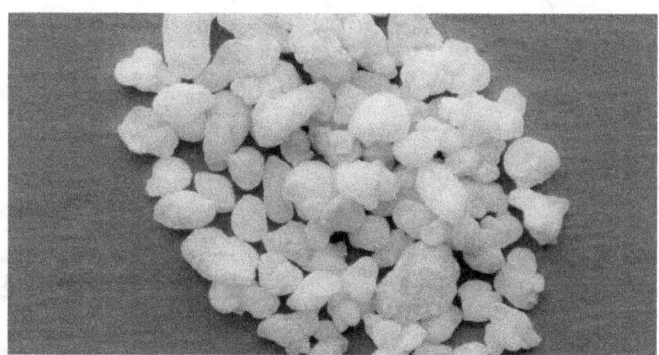

How to Use Frankincense Oil

- Inhaling a few deep breaths of frankincense essential oil will help subdue hunger pangs and induce a calm feeling.

- Add a few drops (2-3) frankincense oil to your diffuser and allow its sweet aroma fill the air surrounding you, this will help to lead away anxious feeling and calm your mind leaving you with lesser cravings.

Jasmine Essential Oil

Jasmine essential oil extracted from the sweet-smelling jasmine bloom, a research study recommends that the scent of Jasmine is very calming.

Jasmine oil has been utilized for quite a long time to cure uneasiness, low sex drive, sleep deprivation and misery; furthermore, research demonstrates that jasmine can calm despondency and elevate your mood.

This trait makes it a phenomenal fundamental oil to use if you are attempting to get in shape and can't control cravings and fell the need to turn to food when you're feeling low or experience difficulty sleeping off at night (which can prompt late night immense consuming of food).

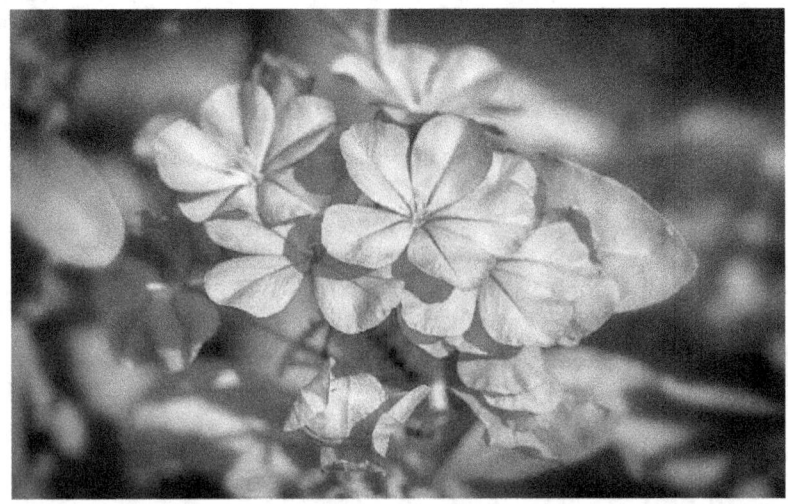

<u>Using Jasmine Essential Oil for Weight Reduction</u>

- Inhale jasmine essential oil before taking a meal, and it will help to calm your senses to prevent you from over-eating. You can also go further to put a few drops of this essential oil on your handkerchief and carry it along with you all day, inhaling from time to time.

- Combine about 2-3 drops of jasmine and about 4-5 drops of grapefruit oil in you diffuse which will send a citrusy scent that will keep you in a good mood and help relax the nerve that causes food cravings.

Orange Essential Oil

Orange oil can control appetite and reduce overeating. It contains Vitamin C and furthermore has a cancer prevention agent benefit. The sharp citrusy aroma is additionally a ground-breaking mood enhancer and can help many experiencing discouragements.A research study from Japan's Mei University demonstrated that orange oil helped members decrease their energizer medicine consumption.

There are uncountable investigations which demonstrate that depression prompts weight increase and this one shows its direct relationship with really causing a higher hazard of obesity

.By utilizing essential oils like orange oil and different oils referenced above, you can lift your mood, feel much improved, and be less enticed to use food to feel better.

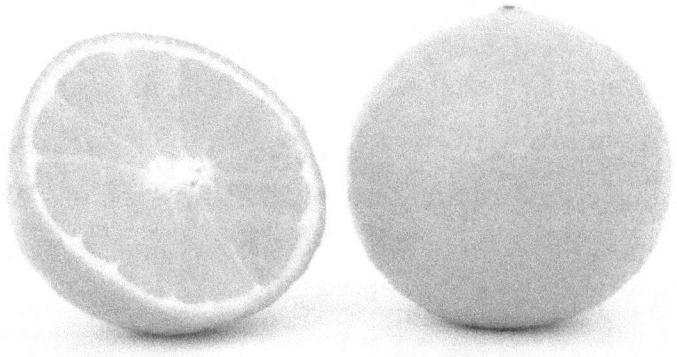

Using Orange Essential Oil for Weight Reduction

- Drink a glass of water containing 1-2 drops of orange oil before you take a meal to help reduce cravings and stop overeating

- Dab a cotton ball in few drops of oil and inhale directly to keep you perked up and stimulate your senses to keep you from overeating.

Rosemary Essential Oil

The rosemary essential oil originates from rosemary sprigs through steam refining. Rosemary essential oil is a solid, ground-breaking oil that can complete something significantly beyond flavor meat and potato dishes.

As indicated by a recent report directed in Japan, rosemary oil can diminish cortisol (the pressure hormone) levels in spit, and this is significant as high cortisol levels relate to dangerous health conditions, for example, hypertension and heart disease.

High cortisol levels lead to elevated feelings of anxiety, which can prompt emotional eating and weight gain. Keeping your cortisol levels low is critical to lessening your feelings of anxiety which will cause less emotional eating and keep your weight in charge.

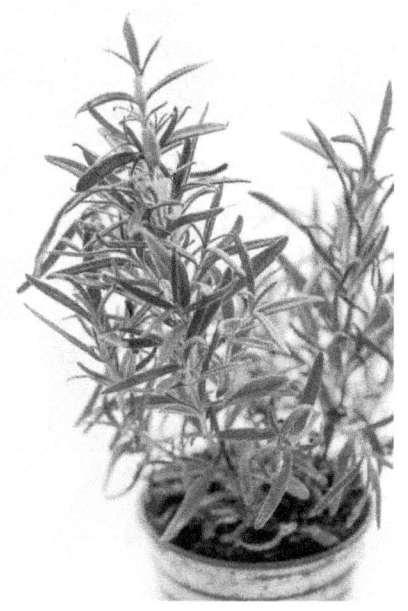

Using Rosemary Essential Oil for Weight Reduction

- When you feel stressed inhale rosemary oil for about 3-5 minutes taking as many deep breaths as you can help in reducing cortisol levels and help your waistline.

Grapefruit Essential Oil:

Grapefruit is well known for helping people lose weight for decades. The grapefruit diet also called the Hollywood Diet since the 1930s.

According to research, when mice are with food containing a lot of fat for three months, the mice were given grapefruit juice to drink gains up to 18% less weight than those that take water.

Grapefruit is gotten from the fresh rind, grapefruit essential oil is an excellent appetite suppressant, detoxifier and helps to prevent water retention in the body and to bloat as it also helps in dissolving fats.

It is a fact that the rind from which the oil originates contains a high concentration of nootkatone, which is a component which is responsible for activating AMP-activated protein kinase (AMPK). AMP-activated protein kinase makes the body reduce fat accumulation and use up sugar which in turn results to weight loss.

In a nutshell, AMP-activated protein kinase is stimulated by grapefruit oil which leads to more fats burned away.In another research, rats are also exposed to grapefruit essential oil 3 times weekly for fifteen minutes, and it led to reduced body weight and food intake in the rats

Limeone is another vital component of grapefruit oil that causes lipolysis (i.e. a process where the body dissolves proteins and fats), this allows reducing appetite and body fat.

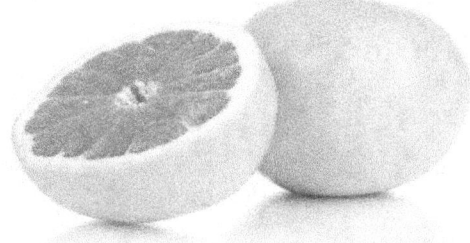

Using Grapefruit Essential Oil for Weight Loss

- Diffuse: put a few drops of grapefruit oil into your diffuser especially when you want to stop late night snacking.

- Dink it: put two drops of therapeutic-grade grapefruit essential oil in water, one glass full. You must ensure that you drink this every morning as soon as you wake up, this will help in increasing the reaction, detoxifying the body by flushing out toxins, increasing fat loss and helps in maintaining your weight.

  After taking a meal, you could also drink the grapefruit oil as it helps to digest food.

- Inhale directly: if suddenly, you are craving, the fresh scent of grapefruit oil can do a lot. You can decide to inhale it directly from a bottle, or you can also add a few drops into a cotton ball and inhale deeply. The scent of grapefruit makes the parasympathetic gastric nerve (the body mechanism that allows ghrelin-induced feeding) to relax.

- Apply topically: you could apply it by rubbing it on your wrist, temples, chest and also under your nose as it helps to curb appetite and also control carvings.

- Reduce cellulite: the oil is also effective in preventing water retention and also activates the lymphatic system. It contains a powerful anti-inflammatory enzyme called bromelain that allows and stimulates the breakdown of cellulite.

  That is why many producers use grapefruit in many cellulite creams. If you want to reduce the cellulite naturally, try the chemical-free blend written below.

Grapefruits Essential Oil All Natural Cellulite Cream:

Ingredients:

15 drops grapefruit oil

Glass Jar

1/2 cup coconut oil

<u>Instructions:</u>

In a blender, blend the coconut oil with the grapefruit oil and store the mixture in a glass jar. Rub onto the part of the skin that has cellulite and massage for 5 minutes daily.

Ginger Essential Oil:

Ginger as an anti-inflammatory is necessary for weight loss as it reduces inflammation which allows a more efficient absorption and digestion of food nutrients.In ginger, a compound called gingerols. Study indicates that this compound called gingerols reduces inflammation in the intestines and therefore makes the overall absorption of nutrients more efficient as it also helps in preventing diseases.

As long as your goal is to lose weight, the ginger essential oil will assist in absorbing the minerals and vitamins that you need to improve your cellular function and energy. You can be sure that it helps you to achieve your weight loss intentions.

A research done in 2013 showed us that ginger oil "possesses antioxidant activity as well as significant anti-inflammatory" properties and in about a month improved enzyme levels in the lab mice's blood had noticeably reduced chronic inflammation.

Another research in 2014 also indicated that to reduce obesity that is caused by increased fat diet, supplementing with ginger will help a great deal. The study also concluded that ginger is a "promising adjuvant therapy for the treatment of obesity."

Ginger oil helps a lot if you are having problems with fat belly. An article published in 2004 in the Biological Pharmaceutical Bulletin indicates that ginger is a cortisol suppressant.

Blood cortisol levels can be caused by High cortisol level which is also as a result of a hormonal imbalance and stressful lifestyle, and this could also push the body's natural metabolism out of place.

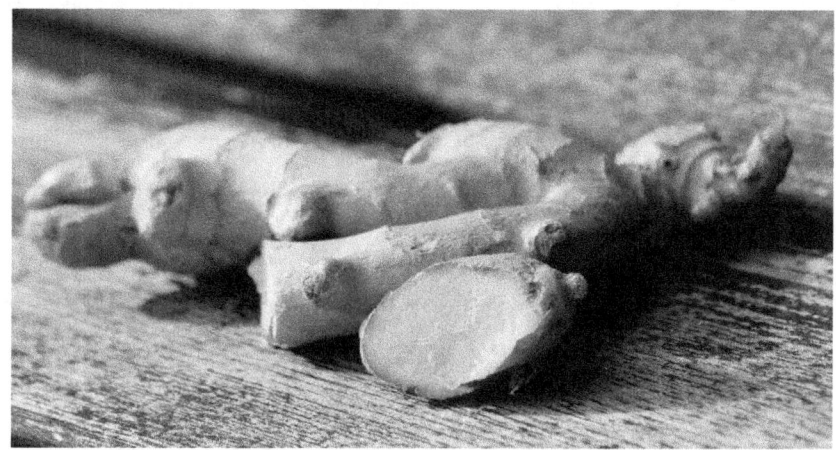

Using Ginger Essential Oil for Weight Loss:

- By drinking it: FDA authorizes that ginger oil has no side effects or dangers when taken directly internally, but it is best and advisable that you use therapeutic-grade ginger oil for internal use. You can also include one to two drops of ginger oil into a warm glass of water and also a squeeze of lemon juice and some honey (raw honey would be advisable).

- Inhale directly: you can also inhale the smell of the ginger oil straight out of the bottle as it serves as a great pick-me-up and also reduces unnecessary appetites and food cravings.

Peppermint Essential Oil

Peppermint has been in use for quite a long time, and it has been used to treat indigestion and particularly when joined with caraway oil has it can help to loosen up stomach muscles and swelling.

The cooling therapeutic compound in peppermint oil, menthol, is phenomenal for improving digestion, expelling gas from the stomach and intestines and easing an irritated stomach.

Menthol can impact neurosensory discernments to change how we taste and smell nourishment, avoiding cravings for sugary sustenances, other sustenance cravings and curbing gorging.

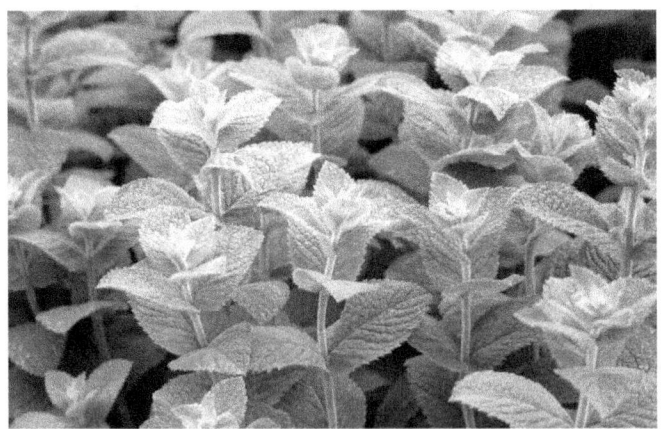

Using Peppermint Essential Oil for Weight Loss:

- Inhale it: You can decide to inhale it directly from a bottle, or you can also add a few drops into a cotton ball and inhale deeply.

The smell of the peppermint can take your mind away from food giving you a sense of relaxation. If you do this before eating, it can help prevent overeating and reduces your appetite.

According to the FDA, it is safe to take internally. About 1 to 2 drops of peppermint essential oil could also be added to a glass of water and taken before a meal as it helps to suppress and reduce appetite.

It is advisable that you buy and use therapeutic grade peppermint essential oil. Therapeutic grade peppermint essential oil is 100% pure and toxin and additives free. You can be rest assured that therapeutic grade peppermint essential oil is undiluted and unfiltered.

- Diffuse: by adding a few drops of peppermint essential oil into your diffuser especially when you feel like snacking. The mint scent is capable of curbing depression and will also go a long way in getting you energized.

Sandalwood Essential Oil

It is also advisable that you eat when you are stressed out if you are an emotional eater. Sandalwood essential oil also helps in reducing depression and creates a sense of calm. It has an exciting woody scent.

It also has a therapeutic effect on that part of the brain that dictates primal emotions like hunger, pleasure, anger and more. It makes a balance in your emotions, and thus food will not be something you turn to feel good. When this is done, you are a step closer to achieving your weight loss goal.

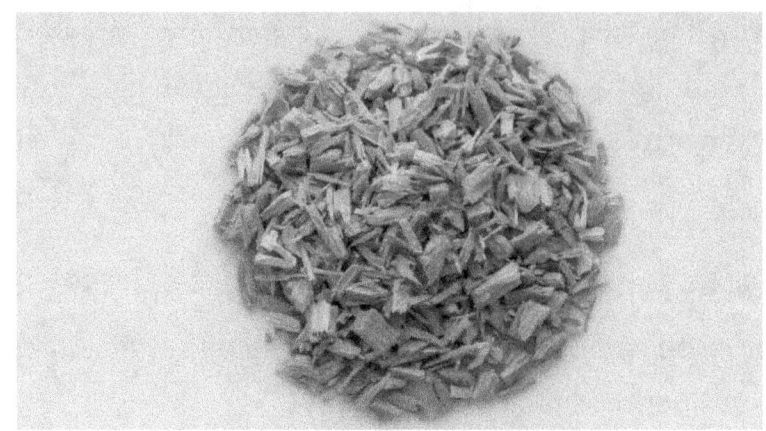

<u>Using Sandalwood Essential Oil for Weight Loss:</u>

- Inhale it: You can decide to inhale it directly from a bottle, or you can also add a few drops into a cotton ball and inhale deeply. The smell of the sandalwood can take your mind away from food giving you a sense of relaxation.

- Apply topically: you could apply it by rubbing it on your wrist and ankle as it helps to curb appetite and also control carvings after a long day's job.

- Diffuse: by adding a few drops of sandalwood essential oil into your diffuser especially when you feel like snacking.

Lavender Essential Oil

Each of the essential oils works in various ways in fighting weight loss. Some works in preventing fat accumulation, some others aids digestion, while others reduce appetite and lots more.

A significant factor that causes obesity today is anxiety and depression. "Feelings such as guilt, sadness, anger, and anxiety can often trigger series of overeating" says the National Centre for Eating Disorder.

Study indicates that stress and anxiety can be calmed by using lavender essential oil. Lavender oil also reduces that trigger that causes emotional eating.

Lavender oil also reduces cortisol level. Cortisols level has to do with the stress hormone that allows the body to retain fat which makes it tougher to lose weight.

A research done in 2010 by International Clinical Pharmacology indicates people using 80 mg per day of lavender showed less anxiety than those using a placebo. Another study done in 2013 shows that when rats are exposed to lavender for seven days inhibited depression-like behaviors and anxiety.

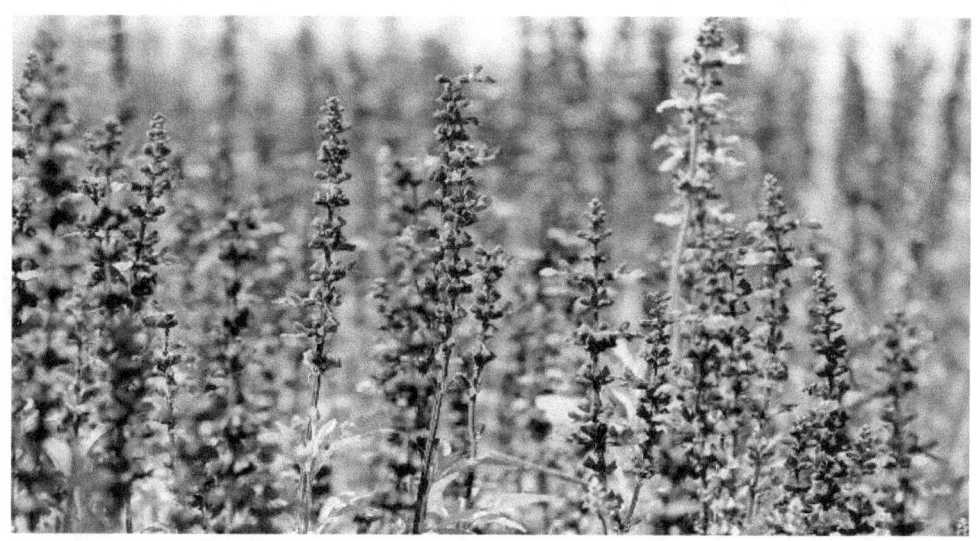

<u>Using Lavender Essential Oil for Weight Loss:</u>

- You can decide to inhale it directly from a bottle, or you can also add a few drops into a cotton ball and inhale deeply.

The fresh scent enters the brain's center of emotion called amygdala and can take your mind away from food giving you a sense of relaxation and by adding a few drops of sandalwood essential oil into your diffuser especially when you feel like snacking.

The pleasant aroma wafts around in the air and helps in reducing food temptation and anxiousness.

Chapter 3 – Essential Oil Recipes for Weight Loss

Weight Loss Capsule

Ingredients:

12 drops fractionated (liquid) coconut oil

2 drops lemon essential oil

2 drops peppermint essential oil

Vegetarian gel capsule (empty)

2 drops grapefruit essential oil

Instructions:

- ✓ Mix the coconut oil with the essential oils in a small container very well.
- ✓ Put the mixture into the capsule using an eyedropper.
- ✓ Use a capsule before breakfast daily to help with weight loss.

More recipes can be used at once to prepare capsule worth a week or even more.

Appetite – Curbing Diffuser Blend

Ingredients:

1 drop spearmint essential oil

3 drops grapefruit essential oil

1 drop ylang-ylang or rose essential oil

3 drops lemon essential oil

Instructions:

- ✓ Mix all the essentials oils in the ingredient list for this recipe in a diffuser.

- ✓ Before having a meal, diffuse one to two hours.

Essential Oil Boosted Drinking Water

Ingredients:

2 liters of drinking water

8 drops grapefruit essential oil

Instructions:

- ✓ Put the grapefruit essential oil into the 2 liters of water.

- ✓ To assist with the weight loss and also to eat less, take the 2 glasses of grapefruit mixed with water an hour or two hours before meal.

Weight Loss Foot Rub

Ingredients:

5 drops cypress essential oil

4 drops lavender essential oil

2 teaspoons carrier oil of choice (argan, avocado, coconut, sesame, sweet almond, jojoba, grapeseed, macadamia)

3 drops juniper essential oil

4 drops basil essential oil

8 drops grapefruit essential oil

Instructions:

- ✓ In a small beaker, mix all the ingredient above.

- ✓ Gently rub on the feet before going to bed (you could add water to increase efforts towards weight loss)

- ✓ You can use More quantity can be used for more than one use.

Weight Loss Massage Oil

Ingredients:

30 drops lemon ESSENTIAL OIL

40 drops grapefruit ESSENTIAL OIL

30 drops rose ESSENTIAL OIL

30 drops geranium ESSENTIAL OIL

1 ounce fractionated (liquid) coconut oil

Instructions:

- ✓ In a glass bottle, mix all of the ingredients above.

- ✓ Use it on your body taking your while taking bathing to help speed up weight loss, and you could use a professional massage session.

Citrus Anti-Cellulite Cream

Ingredients:

2 tablespoons witch hazel

10 drops lemon essential oil

30 drops grapefruit essential oil

¾ cup of coconut oil

2 tablespoons beeswax

Instructions:

- ✓ In a small bowl, mix the essential oils with the witch hazel.

- ✓ In a double boiler using medium heat, dissolve the beeswax and the coconut oil making sure that they melt.

- ✓ When you complete the above, remove from heat and mix the oils with witch hazel then stir gently to mix thoroughly.

- ✓ Put the result of the above step in a glass jar and wait to cool.

- ✓ Cover the glass tightly and store in a cool place. Wait for about 3 hours before making use.

Better Than a Tummy Tuck Cream

Ingredients:

15 drops geranium ESSENTIAL OIL

¼ cup beeswax (grated)

15 drops lavender ESSENTIAL OIL

15 drops grapefruit ESSENTIAL OIL

1 cup extra virgin olive oil

15 drops frankincense ESSENTIAL OIL

⅛ cup vitamin E oil

1 cup rose water

Instructions:

- ✓ In a double boiler, add all the ingredients above apart from the rose water and the essential oils.

- ✓ Place the mixture on medium heat until all the ingredients melt.

- ✓ Place the result into a blender and allow it to cool

- ✓ When you do this, blend the result until it is all thoroughly mixed (scrap the sides as you go).

- ✓ As you keep on blending, gently add the rose water to emulsify the mixture.

- ✓ Add also all the essential oil and blend quickly to incorporate them into the mixture.

- ✓ Add the cream into the glass jar and tightly cover it.

- ✓ Apply it daily on the abdomen to tighten the skin and reduce fat.

Chapter 4 – What to Look Out For When Buying Essential Oils?

It is vital that when you are buying essential oils, ensure that the bottle says '100% pure essential oil'. Also, make sure that the correct name of the species is well indicated in the label of the bottle.

If the word 'fragrance' is seen, have it in mind that there are almost always other additives.It is advisable that you buy essential oils from an organic source labelled as 'Therapeutic grade', this shows that they are toxin and additive free.

Therapeutic grades are undiluted and unfiltered. Be warned not to choose from Non-Genetically Modified Ingredients.

Conclusion

Closing Tips for Using Essential Oils to Achieve Your Weight Loss Goals

If you are a beginner to using essential oils, here are a few things that you should know to ease using them.

Firstly, it is advisable that if you are using essential oil as a newbie, ensure you do a body patch test on a small part of your skin (advisably your arm or leg) before you apply it on your whole body by rubbing or taking it directly internally. When you complete, whether you are allergic to an oil or not would be detected before you use a higher number of dosage.

Essential oils that pass this first quick skin patch test may be mildly irritating when you use them directly. You can also dilute your oil in a carrier oil like olive oil, coconut oil or jojoba oil before using it directly on your skin.

Ensure you limit the use of citrus-based oils (like orange and lemon essential oil) before using long period time outdoors, particularly during pool season and beach because they can be a cause of phototoxicity

Many oils are for external use only although it is not harmful if taken internally. But also make sure you get them fit for consumption before ingesting it.Lastly, always aim for the highest grade of essential oil that you can get.

Essential oils are implemented in various ways which are:

- ✓ capsules

- ✓ bath and body products

- ✓ massage oil

- ✓ diffusion

- ✓ rubs and balms

- ✓ inhalation

- ✓ food and drink recipes (when safe for internal use)

To achieve your weight loss goal, any of the recipes written above would apply. You can also take some recipes along with you to school, recreational activities, travel and work by making portable recipes. Your bracelet and necklace can be made with ceramic diffuser beads to hold the scent of your essential oil all day.

Essential oil isn't a miracle, they are only a push to your weight loss efforts. Don't stop your medication or prescription provided by your doctor. Using essential oil also shouldn't be a reason for living a reckless diet lifestyle.

Furthermore, problems such as depression, digestive disorder, autoimmune disorders, hypothyroidism and anxiety and other health and mood related issues associated with weight can be addressed using essential oils.

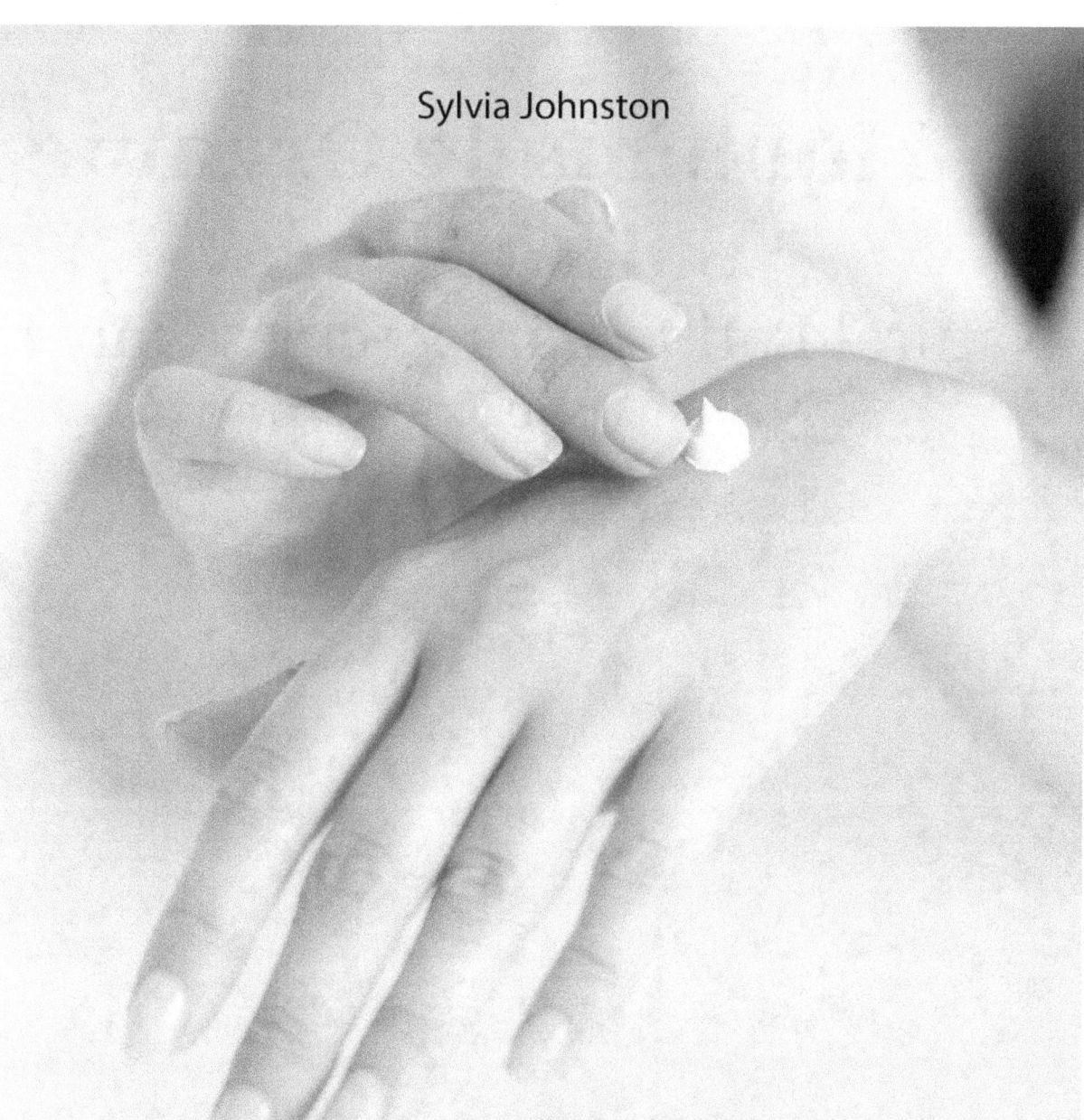

Sylvia Johnston

HOMEMADE ORGANIC LOTION BARS:

Natural Lotion Bars Recipes
Only from Non-Toxic Ingredients

Homemade Organic Lotion Bars:

Natural Lotion Bars Recipes Only from Non-Toxic Ingredients

Introduction: Quality that Can't Be Store Bought

Quality homemade bars of soap loaded with non-toxic all-natural ingredients such as lemon, citrus, and coconut are of a higher caliber than most of their store-bought brethren.

And drop in a few special oil-based compounds such as soybean oil, jasmine, or rosemary and you've got yourself a real winning combination. These DIY soaps cleanse as well as they soothe, and provide an unbeatable fragrance. All while providing you a way to cut off the daily bombardment of toxic chemicals that regular soap users are routinely exposed to.

So, if you are looking for a book to provide you with some wholesome soap recipes with all-natural ingredients, then look no further. Because this book, and the soap recipes herein, provide the kind of quality that just can't be store bought.

Chapter 1: Getting Your Soapy Supplies Ready

Soap making is a rich and rewarding experience but its only going to work if you have the right supplies. Besides the actual ingredients for your soap, you will need things like soap molds, protective gear, and appropriate cooking utensils. Here in this chapter we will give you a brief overview to get your soapy supplies ready!

Protective Goggles

As you work with soap it would be a good idea to where some sort of protective goggles. Although soap may seem like a tame enough material, there are chemicals involved, and any time you work with chemicals you run the risk of irritation to your eyes. Lye for example, can be particularly dangerous if it gets into your eyes.

The best way to avoid this danger is to simply make sure that your eyes are protected and covered at all times. They should be protected in this fashion during the whole process of soap making.

Work Gloves

As good as soap is you see, it is composed of a little something called "alkalies" and since these alkalies have a tremendous ability to dry out and dissolve oil based elements, being exposed to too much of it, or to a densely concentrated form can cause the skin to dry out or even break out into a rash

This is why it is necessary to take preventative measures such as this. Your hands are precious. They are the instruments with which you make your soap so you want to make sure that you protect them! In order to do so you will need to get some thick, industrial class work gloves.

Some may try to make soap with plastic or latex gloves, but these are not good options since borax and lye may eat right through them! Be sure to get some good work gloves!

Dust Mask

Making soap involves a lot of vapors and fumes, so unless you are exceptionally good at holding your breath—I would advise you to wear a protective dust mask. These small, but durable half masks, fit right on your face and serv to keep any wayward components of your soap from finding their way inside your respiratory tract!

And even if you do not suffer from devastating breathing difficulty there are many who have suffered through some pretty bad headaches from lingering fumes, so be sure to cover your face with a proper dust mask before making your soap.

Vinegar

If you have nothing else to use as a hardening agent, a little bit of vinegar could truly do some wonders. For anyone using vinegar, you will need to use just enough to offset the amount of oil that you use. The general rule is to make sure that you are able to replace water and oil with vinegar substrate.

If you do not want to use a whole lot of water, there are many recipes in which you could actually replace at least half of your H2O content with simple, plain old vinegar. As such, be sure to have a couple bottles of vinegar in stock.

Lye

While lye is most certainly not necessary when it comes to making natural soap, it doesn't hurt to have some on hand just in case you might need. Lye can almost be substituted for other oil-based ingredients but there are certain formulas that could use the kick that only lye could provide. Although not mandatory in its use, lye has been a part of soap making for quite a long time.

And there is a reason for its use as an ingredient. Lye is a great binding material and can really bring all of the elements of your soap ingredients together. Be sure to have this and all of the items, and supplies mentioned in this chapter on hand as you go about your soap making process.

Chapter 2: Medicinal and Cleansing Soap

No matter what may be ailing you—sometimes the best medicine you could ever be prescribed is simply a bar of soap that will get you nice and clean. Here in this chapter we provide you with several soapy examples that will do just that!

Almond Cleansing Soap

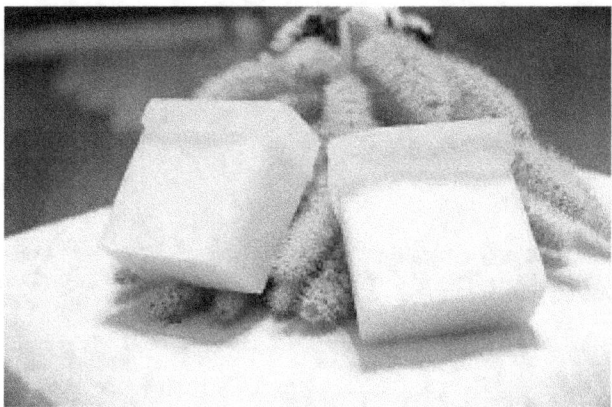

Almonds have a nourishing effect on skin and can bring moisture back to even the driest of surface layers. Almonds after all are full of Vitamin E and as such can provide some extra special protection from such things as the sun's grating rays. Almond soap also has vitamin A which is also quite good at clearing up just about any complexion.

Here are the exact ingredients:

16 ounces of palm oil

22 ounces of soybean oil

7 ounces of coconut oil

5 ounces of almond oil

3 cups of water

To begin, get out a large pot and add your 3 cups of water inside. Now set your stove for medium-high heat. Next, add your 5 ounces of almond oil, your 7 ounces of coconut oil, and your 22 ounces of soybean oil. Stir these a few minutes before adding in your 16 ounces of palm oil. Stir all of your ingredients together well and cook for 10 minutes.

After your ten minutes have passed, turn the stove off, and let the ingredients settle a moment, before you pour the contents of the pot inside the appropriate soap molds of your choosing. Allow the molds to dry out for 15 hours and your soaps are ready for use. You should have enough material to make several bars of soap with.

Organic Scalp Cleansing Soap

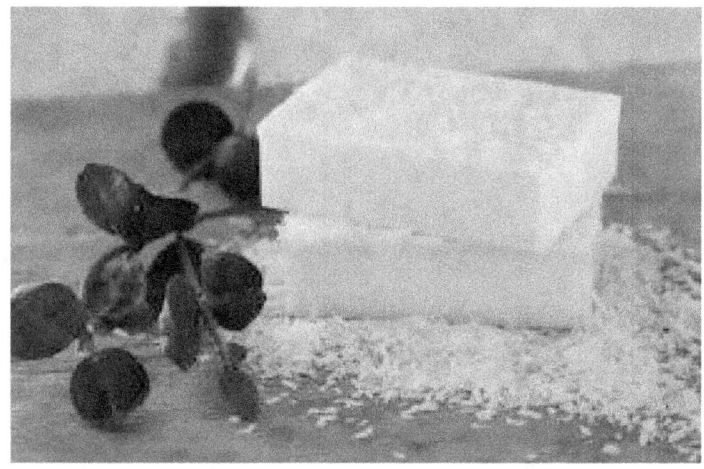

Do you ever have problems with greasy hair or dandruff? Are you looking for an all-natural, organic solution to your itchy scalp? Well then you should most certainly give this Organic Scalp Cleansing Soap a try!

I can remember times that my hair was so flaky I thought it was snowing every time I brushed it! But after just a few weeks of using this very special soap, my hair soon became free of dandruff and a whole lot less oily. This DIY soap delight is highly recommended.

Here are the exact ingredients:

3 ounces of lye

4 ounces of cocoa butter

4 ounces of coconut oil

3 ounces of castor oil

3 ounces of jojoba oil

3 ounces of Shea butter

2 ounces of beeswax

4 ounces of coconut milk

2 cups of water

First, get out a mixing bowl and deposit your 2 ounces of lye, your 2 cups of water, and your 4 ounces of coconut milk inside.Stir these ingredients together well before pouring them into a pan. Set your stove on medium-high heat and stir the ingredients continually over the next 15 to 20 minutes.

Now get out an additional mixing bowl and add your 2 ounces of beeswax, your 3 ounces of Shea butter, your 3 ounces of jojoba oil, your 3 ounces of castor oil, and your 4 ounces of coconut oil. Stir these ingredients together well and put the mixing bowl in the microwave on high heat for about 30 seconds. The ingredients should melt and meld together well.

After this, dump the melted mixing bowl ingredients into the pan on the stove, stir everything together and cook on medium-high heat for another few minutes.

Finally, pour the cooked ingredients into your soap molds and let them dry and solidify within the mold for 15 hours.

The Veggie Cleanser

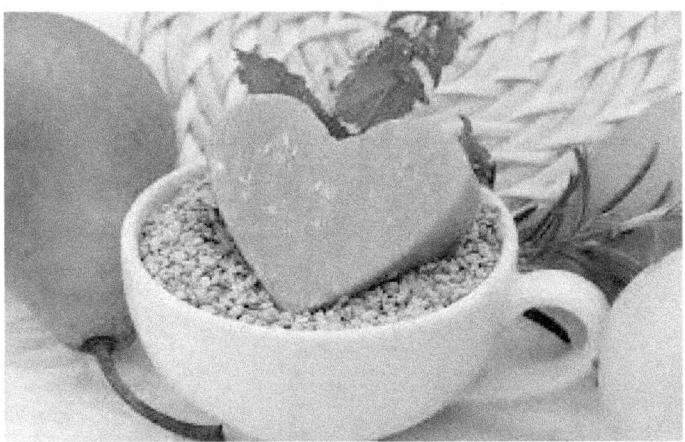

Remember when your folks told you to eat your vegetables? Well what about washing with them? Vegetable soap? Who would have thought right?But as it turns out the vegetable extracts in this soap bar make for the perfect cleanser! The vitamins and nutrients in this soap are just perfect for rebuilding degenerative tissue of the skin. This is regenerative (and clean) medicine at its best!

Here are the exact ingredients:

18 ounces of carrot juice

20 ounces of coconut oil

18 ounces of canola oil

18 ounces of vegetable oil

20 ounces of olive oil

3 cups of water

To begin, place a pot on the stove, set the temp for medium-high and then add your 3 cups of water to the pot. After this add your 18 ounces of carrot juice followed by your 20 ounces of coconut oil, your 18 ounces of canola oil, your 18 ounces of vegetable oil, and your 20 ounces of olive oil.

Now stir everything together as it cooks over the next 15 to 20 minutes. Finally, take your cooked ingredients and pour them into some molds. Allow them to harden for about 10 hours before use.

Medicinal Lavender

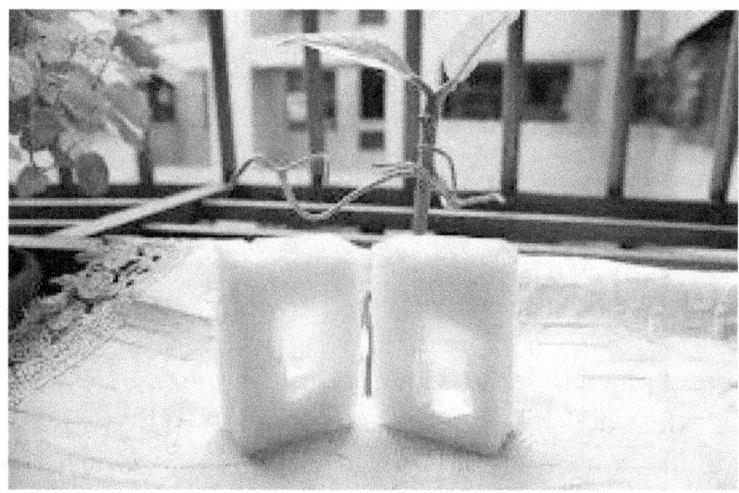

Lavender has many medicinal properties such as being able to ease inflammation. As such, this soap can work wonders for someone who has broken out into a rash.

I can personally vouch for this due to a run in with some poison ivy earlier this spring. I was doing some yard work when I came into contact with the toxic plant and both of my arms broke out as a result.But by scrubbing away at the inflamed skin with some good old Medicinal Lavender I was able to take much of the sting out of the poison ivy rash and speed up my recovery.

If you are having skin issues, you never have to suffer in silence again. Just make this soap bar and make it a part of your daily routine. You'll be glad that you did. This soap is highly recommended.

Here are the exact ingredients:

1 ounce of almond oil

1 ounce of palm oil

1 ounce of coconut oil

4 ounces of lavender oil

2 ounces of olive oil

3 cups of milk

1 cup of water

Get out a pot and place it onto a stove set for high heat. Now add your 3 cups of milk and 1 cup of water to the pot. This should then be followed by your ounce of almond oil, your ounce of palm oil, your ounce of coconut oil, and your 2 ounces of olive oil.

Briefly stir these ingredients before adding your 4 ounces of lavender oil. Now mix it all up and allow to cook for about 30 minutes. After this pour the mixture directly into your molds and have them solidify and dry out over the next 10 hours.

Chapter 3: Non-Toxic Cosmetic Soap

There are a lot of toxins in our normal everyday environment, and surprisingly many of the store-bought soaps, shampoos, and deodorants have more than their fair share of toxins as well. It does seem rather ironic that we would lather up and wash ourselves with something that contains toxins, but this is actually standard fare for most.

Having that said, it's really no wonder people have dry skin, flaky, dandruff filled hair, and inflamed armpits. In order to break away from this detrimental routine, here in this chapter we present to you some of the best DIY recipes for non-toxic cosmetic soap.

Banana Boat Soap

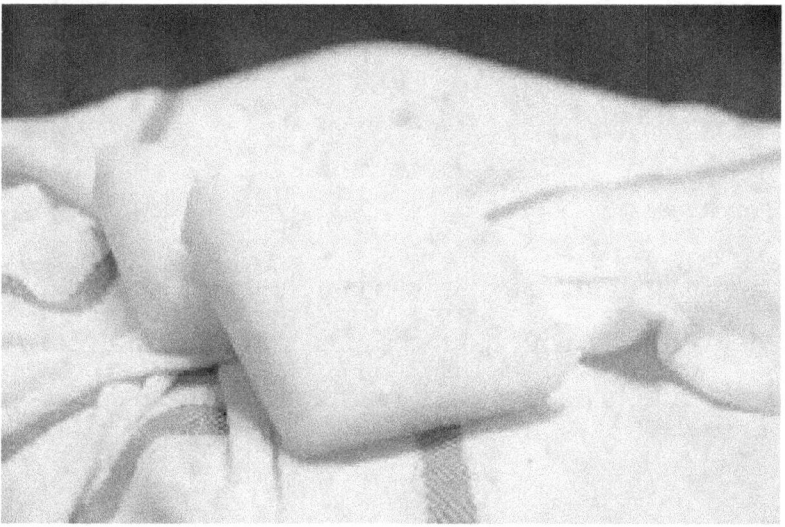

You like Bananas? Then you are going to love this soap! This banana-based soap does a tremendous job of moisturizing and cleansing your skin. It's a dual-purpose workhorse of clean goodness at your disposal.

The main ingredient of this soap—potassium hydroxide—is excellent at evenly distributing moisture throughout the cells of the skin as well as balancing out the entire PH level of the dermis.

Here are the exact ingredients:

4 ounces of borax

5 ounces of potassium hydroxide

5 ounces of coconut oil

10 ounces of olive oil

2 cups of water

To get started, get out a large pot and place it on a stove adjusted for medium-high heat. Now add your 2 cups of water to the pot and wait a few minutes until the water comes to a boil.

Once the water is beginning to boil you can then add your 4 ounces of borax, your 5 ounces of potassium hydroxide, your 5 ounces of coconut oil, and your 10 ounces of olive oil. Stir all of these ingredients together well for about 15 minutes.

Once your 15 minutes have passed you can then pour your ingredients into your waiting soap molds and allow them to solidify into hard bars of soap over the next 10 hours.

Exfoliating Lemon Bar

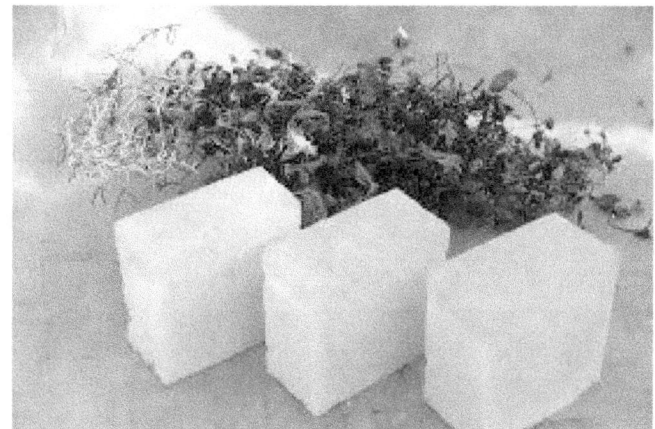

Have you ever noticed how so many cleaning products from laundry detergent to dish soap are either "lemon scented" or otherwise have lemon as a main ingredient? There is indeed a reason for this Lemon you see, is a natural cleaning agent. This soap cleans, exfoliates, and leaves you with a fresh lemony scent! And this soap in particular is fantastic at scraping away the grime and leaving you clean and fresh!

Here are the exact ingredients:

11 ounces of lemon juice

1 ounce of lemon oil

1 cup of water

1 cup of milk

In order to create your own exfoliating lemon bar, you will need to get out a large pot and add your cup of water and your cup of milk to the pot. Stir these ingredients together for a few minutes and allow to come to a boil.

After this, you can then add your 11 ounces of lemon juice, and your ounce of lemon oil. Stir these ingredients together well over the course of the next 8 to 10 minutes. Once thoroughly mixed and cooked, you can then pour the mixture into soap molds. Allow the soaps to solidify over the next 10 hours.

Orange Face Soap

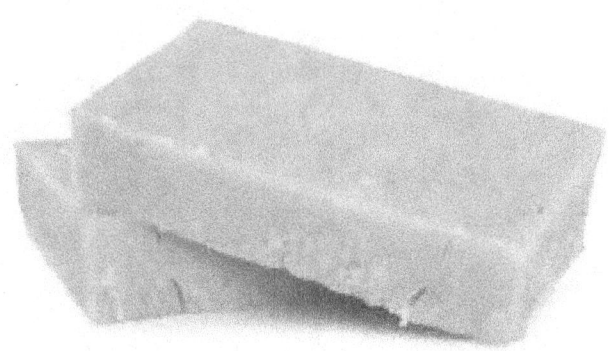

Despite what the Oompa Loompas may have told you this soap doesn't mean you'll have an orange face after using it! The soap itself is made out of orange juice, along with special infused oils, and cocoa butter. Orange juice is a natural exfoliating and the exfoliating element that it provides in this soap is nothing short of tremendous.

This soap can naturally rejuvenate the skin and provide relief from blemishes. If for example you are suffering from acne, or even eczema—this soap could be of tremendous help in your recovery. Oranges are a medicinal food that help boost our immune system and they provide relief to inflammation. This soap is a real winner. You are really going to love it!

Here are the exact ingredients:

12 ounces of orange juice

1 ounce of orange oil

5 ounces of olive oil

4 ounces of cocoa butter

2 cups of water

Orange bar soap is great for the skin and is as nourishing as it is enriching. In order to create your own orange bar soap fill cup a large pot with 2 cups of water and place it on a stove set for medium-high heat.

Next, add your 12 ounces of orange juice, your ounce of orange oil, your 5 ounces of olive oil and your 4 ounces of cocoa butter. Stir and cook these ingredients over the next 10 minutes. Once your 10 minutes have passed you can then pour your soap mixture into your soap molds and leave them out to dry for about 15 hours.

Palm Kernel Shave Cream Soap

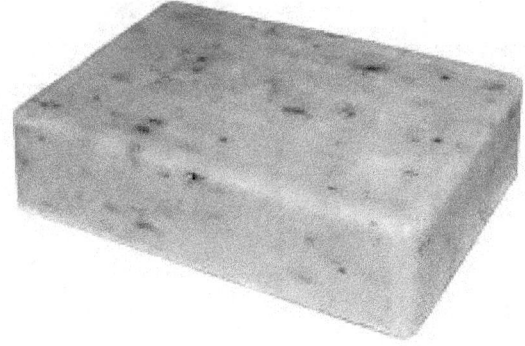

Palm Kernel Shave Cream Soap! Good for your face, arms, legs, armpits—or whatever else you may have to shave! The all-natural chemistry of this soap really comes together to create a smooth glide for your razor blade. With this mixture of coconut and palm kernel, it's always a real pleasure to lather up for a close shave.

Here are the exact ingredients:

10 ounces of palm kernel oil

10 ounces of olive oil

5 ounces of coconut oil

1 cup of water

To produce this rich soap, start off with a medium sized pan and a cup of water. Next, add in your 10 ounces of palm kernel oil and your 10 ounces of olive oil followed by your 5 ounces of coconut oil.

Stir these ingredients together well as they cook over the next 5 minutes. Once thoroughly mixed together you can then pour the mix into your soap molds. Allow to harden for at least 8 hours before use.

Chapter 4: Soap for Your Pets

Anyone who has a cat or dog know just how difficult grooming your animals can be. They don't like the water, and they don't like the soap. They would rather be anywhere but where you are when it's for them to wash up.

But washing your pets does not have to be a terrible chore. The homemade soaps presented in this chapter provide a tremendous resource to all of your pet cleaning efforts. If you need a good soap for your pet feel free to try them all.

Dog Gone Soap

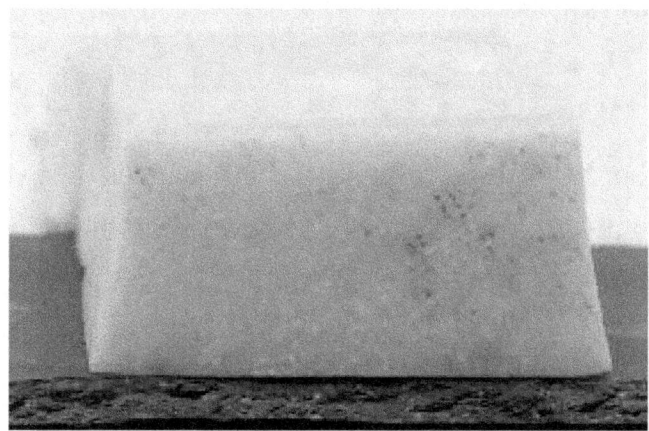

If your doggie needs a good soap to get him up and going. You might want to give this one a try. It's loaded with soybean and olive oil. This recipe creates just the right mixture to keep the moisture in your dog's scalp but out of its hair. This soap is also a tremendous oil fighter, providing your dog with a great clean coat of fur.

Here are the exact ingredients:

3 ounces of soybean oil

3 ounces of olive oil

3 ounces of coconut oil

3 ounces of avocado oil

4 ounces of rosemary oil

1 ounce of lye

2 cups of water

Put your 2 cups of water into a pot, followed by your ounce of lye. Set the stove for high heat. Now stir the ingredients together as they cook a few minutes before adding in your 3 ounces of avocado oil.

Stir these together briefly and then add your 3 ounces of soybean oil, your 3 ounces of olive oil, and your 4 ounces of rosemary oil. Stir and cook these ingredients together for another few minutes. Once everything is mixed and cooked, pour ingredients into soap molds and allow to settle in place for about 8 hours. After this, the soap is ready for use.

Kitty Cat Bar

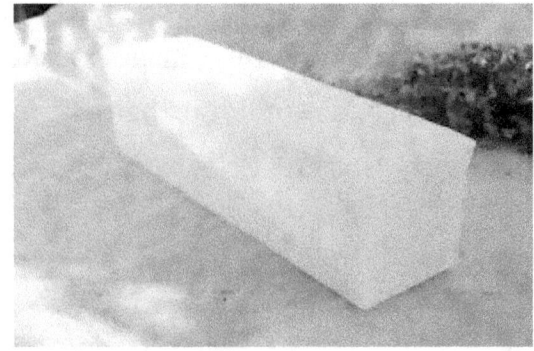

This is some pretty heavy-duty soap for your cat. It's composed primarily of Shea butter, giving it a very smooth sheen. If your cat needs an extra shine to its coat you may want to give this Kitty Cat Bar a try.

Here are the exact ingredients:

4 ounces of Shea butter

4 ounces of beeswax

4 ounces of coconut oil

2 cups of water

Place a large pot onto a stove set for high heat and then add your 2 cups of water. After your water has been added you can then go ahead and add your 4 ounces of Shea butter, your 4 ounces of beeswax, and your 4 ounces of coconut oil.

Stir these ingredients together as they cook over the next few minutes. Turn burner off and allow ingredients to settle in place for a moment before pouring the mixture into your molding. Allow soap mixture to solidify and harden in the soap molds for about 8 hours before use.

Flea and Tick Proof Soap

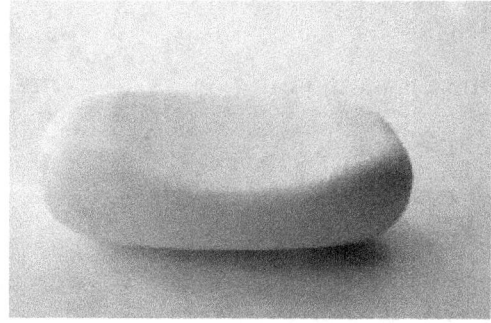

Tick season is terrible this year. I can attest to that myself. The other day I was out in the back of my property walking my dog when I noticed a tick right on top of the little guy's head. It thankfully hadn't attached yet so I went to knock it off. Right after knocking this tick off I then noticed another one crawling on my arm!

I think both me and my dog both were ready to run inside at that point! But the best way to beat the ticks this season is simply to stay as clean as possible. After your dog comes in from a long excursion outdoors wash him down with this flea and tick proof soap and those critters won't stand a chance.

Here are the exact ingredients:

3 cups of cinnamon oil

3 cups of thyme

3 cups of clove oil

4 cups of rosemary

3 cups of beeswax

3 cups of mango butter

1 cup of coconut oil

2 cups of water

To get started, deposit your 2 cups of water into a pot and set the stove for high heat. Now add your 3 cups of cinnamon oil, your 3 cups of thyme, your 3 cups of clove oil, your 4 cups of rosemary, your 3 cups of beeswax, your 3 cups of mango butter, and your cup of coconut oil.

Stir everything together well as they cook over the course of the next ten minutes. After this, pour the mixture into your molds and allow them to harden for the next 10 hours. Once hardened, use when ready.

Furry Friend Fragrance

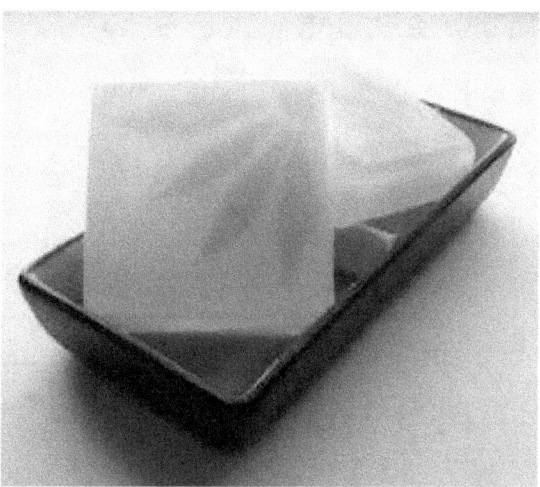

If your little doggy has been smelling kind of funny lately, you just might want to give him a little bit of help in the odor apartment.

Many dog soaps simply mask the odor but the great thing about this fragrant bit of soap is that it neutralizes the odor at the source as well as leaving a fragrant aroma behind in its wake. Don't let your dog stink! Give him the Furry Friend Fragrance he needs!

Here are the exact ingredients:

3 ounces of citronella

3 ounces of sweet orange essential oil

5 ounces of coconut oil

14 ounces of olive oil

5 ounces of lye

2 cups of water

Making this soap is a breeze. Simply get out a large pot, place onto a stove at medium-high heat, and add your 2 cups of water. After this, you can then add your 3 ounces of citronella, your 3 ounces of sweet orange essential oil, your 5 ounces of coconut oil, your 14 ounces of olive oil, and finally your 5 ounces of lye.

Stir these ingredients together well over the course of the next 20 minutes. Once cooked allow to settle in the pot for a moment before pouring into your molding. Keep the soap mixture inside your molding for about 10 hours. Once hard and dry, this soap is ready for use.

Chapter 5: Uniquely Made Soap Creations

Have you ever heard of soap made out of Dr. Pepper? What about beer? Yes, sometimes it seems that soap can be literally made out of just about anything, and here in this chapter we show you some truly unique homemade soap creations.

The Budweiser Bar

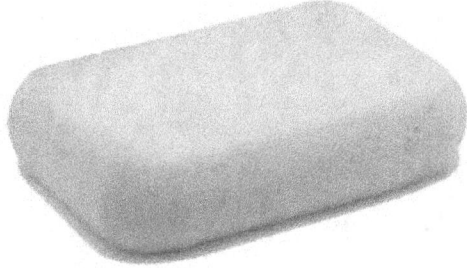

Rather than drinking Budweiser at the bar why not take a bat with a Budweiser bar of soap! Before you think this is absolutely batty just consider the fact that beer is a great cleanser and exfoliant for the skin!

Yep, that's right! Studies have actually proven that the hops component of common, everyday beer is full of all kinds of enriching amino acids that make the skin smooth and soft!

Beer actually has a lot of skin healthy vitamins as well, making it an all-around skin friendly cocktail of ingredients! And don't worry—this soap won't keep you from driving home afterwards!

Here are the exact ingredients:

30 ounces of Budweiser

10 ounces of olive oil

10 ounces of coconut oil

1 cup of water

In order to make your own Budweiser soap, get out a large pot, put it on a stove set for medium-high heat and add your cup of water. Next add your 30 ounces of Budweiser, followed by your 10 ounces of olive oil, and your 10 ounces of coconut oil.

Stir these ingredients together well over the next 10 minutes. Turn your stove off and allow the mixture to settle for a minute or so. After this, you can then pour the mixture into your molding. Keep inside the soap molds for at least 8 hours. They should now be solid and ready for use.

Soda Bar Soap

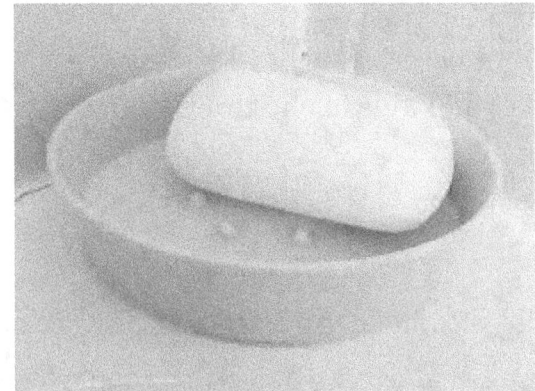

Would you like to try some soda soap? No—we're not talking baking soda here—we're talking soda soda! Made from any variety of soda-based beverage you could imagine, this novelty soap is not only unique, it actually cleans pretty good too! Even while allowing you to smell like grape soda! Isn't life great?

Here are the exact ingredients:

20 ounces of a soda-based beverage

10 ounces of lemon juice

2 ounces of borax

2 cups of water

Get out a large cooking pot and add your 2 cups of water before setting the stovetop burner to medium heat. Now add your 20 ounces of soda (Dr. Pepper, Pepsi, any beverage you like), followed by your 10 ounces of lemon juice, and your 2 ounces of borax. Take especial care to keep the borax out of your eyes, as it can cause irritation.

Stir everything together well and cook for about 3 to 5 minutes. After this, let the mixture settle a bit before pouring into your soap molds. Keep the mixture in the soap molds over the next 8 to 10 hours. They should now be ready to be pried out of the molding. Use whenever you are ready to do so.

Spicy Soap

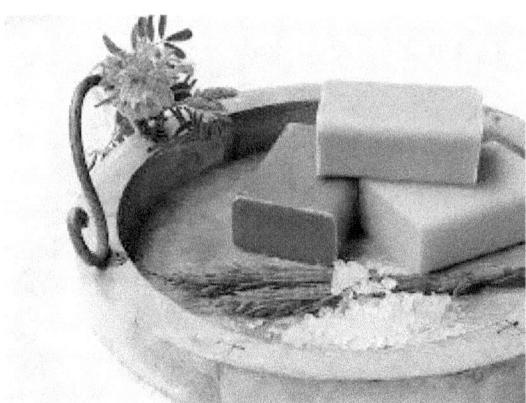

If you want to add some spice in your nice and cleanly life, add this Spicy Soap to your bath time regimen! This soap dares to include 10 full ounces of habanero oil. Habanero oil you see is full of a little something called curcumin. Curcumin is good for us in a wide variety of ways from fighting inflammation to slowing down our metabolism.

In soap form it is its inflammation fighting power that is the most promising. Just lather up some of this skin on an arm broken out in a rash and soon enough that arm will be as clear as the day you were born! This soap is also an excellent exfoliant and quite good at clearing up acne. Go ahead and give this Spicy Soap a try! You will most certainly be glad that you did!

Here are the exact ingredients:

10 ounces of habanero oil

2 ounces of mango butter

5 ounces of olive oil

5 ounces of coconut oil

2 ounces of lye

1 cup of water

Place a large pot onto your stovetop and set the burner on high. Add your cup of water followed by your 10 ounces of habenero oil, your 2 ounces of mango butter, your 5 ounces of olive oil, your 5 ounces of coconut oil, and your 2 ounces of lye.

Stir everything together well over the course of the next 5 to 10 minutes. Once the mixture has been cooked allow to settle for a moment, and then pour it all out inside of your soap moldings. Keep in moldings for at least 8 hours before use.

Strawberry and Cream Bar

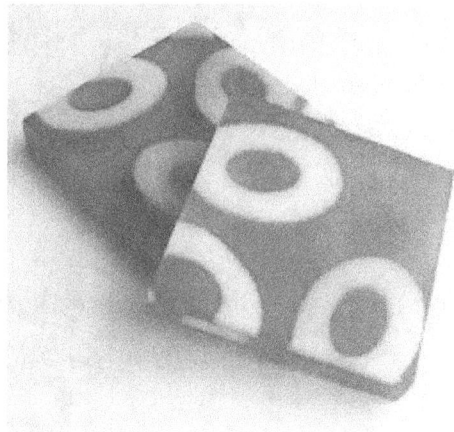

It's like desert decided to pay your bath time routine a visit! What can I say? If you like strawberries and cream then you are going to love this bar of soap! It's more than just a novel luxury however, this soap can really clean and detox your skin!

Strawberry juice is known to slow the aging process of our skin, fighting wrinkles and evening out our skin tone when we get older. The combination of strawberry and coconut are also powerful in antioxidants, greatly boosting the elastic integrity of our dermis. Try this soap today!

Here are the exact ingredients:

7 ounces of strawberry juice

2 ounces of sodium hydroxide

5 ounces of palm oil

5 ounces of coconut oil

3 ounces of lye

2 cups of water

This most certainly is an interesting batch of soap. In order to create your own version— here's what you have to do. Get out a large pot and place it onto a stovetop burner set for high heat. Next, add your 2 cups of water followed by your 7 ounces of strawberry juice, your 2 ounces of sodium hydroxide, your 5 ounces of coconut oil, and your 3 ounces of lye.

Stir everything together well before allowing to settle for 2 or 3 minutes. Finally, pour the mix into your soap molds and let harden for 8 to 10 hours. Once hard and dry, this soap is ready for use!

Conclusion: Where there is Hope—There is Soap!

We see our soap in the soap dish or hanging at the corner rim of our bath tub and not think much of it. But without soap life would be pretty miserable, pretty quickly. Just think of the last time that you really needed nothing more than a hot shower and a good bar of soap.

Maybe you just got back from a long day at work or you were working hard out in the yard—either way, when you were done you knew that nothing would quite make you feel better other than cleaning and refreshing that outside layer we commonly call our skin, with a nice bar of soap.

Soap cleanses, refreshes and heals. And as such, many varieties of soap with many purported purposes have been created throughout the years. Here in this book we have presented to you quite a wide variety of soap types which all have a multiplicity of uses I really do hope that you have find the tips, recipes, and advice in this book helpful.

And if you follow the guidelines of this book as presented to you, I know that this hope is not in vain. Because where there is hope after all—there is soap!

Thank you for reading! And good luck!

Essential Oils For Beginners:

Best Guide To Get Started With Aromatherapy
and Organic Recipes With Essential Oils

Ella Witt

Essential Oils For Beginners

Best Guide To Get Started With Aromatherapy and Organic Recipes With Essential Oils

Introduction

Since the ancient times it is known that essential oils are very beneficial to our overall health. Before we experienced the advancement of modern medicine, essential oils are already present because they are already been used by our forefathers in several purposes.

When it comes to ingredients you will not find any flaws on them because they are completely all-natural or in other words they are a product of different herbs that are combined together to become worthy of your attention.

Before I was really skeptical about it because I thought how come will an essential oil cure such ailments? I tried several ways on how to cure my asthma but did not find any answer even on the medicines that the doctor is giving me that's why, what I did is to go for alternative medicines. This is where I came across the so-called essential oils, I did not knew that it will take a lot of effect on my overall health in a positive way.

To tell you frankly, my problem with my asthma has been completely resolved. I was really shocked with the results because I did not expect that a natural way of healing will suffice the need to cure my chronic condition.

Within a few days, my chronic condition got healed which made me feel happy because I felt a lot of relief. This is the primary reason why I decided to create a book that tackles the different essential oils that you can utilize to help you with your dilemmas.

I personally tried these recipes and they are really effective that's why you are in good hands because you have the peace of mind that it will work and you do not need to experiment anymore because I experimented them and tried it myself.

So by imparting these recipes with you, I have this joy of sharing and at the same time helping you to become overall well. Do not worry because all of the essential oils that we will tackle here are completely safe to use. And as a matter of fact I did not experience any allergic reactions from them.

As you will notice in the following chapters there are essential oils that are repeated because they have more than one use. It is the fact because herbal medicines are proven to target more than one condition.

Do not worry because it does not mean that if you are using an essential oil it tells that you have sickness because essential oils can be used for various purposes which we will discuss further in this book. So brace yourselves as we dive deeper into the different essential oils and their corresponding uses.

Chapter 1 – Essential Oil Recipes For Stress and Anxiety

Stress is prevalent nowadays and became a part of our day to day existence here on the planet. It is an immediate action of our body to combat the threats that we have either negative or not. The dilemma happens when stress stays longer than usual, which results in depression and other types of mental illnesses.

The Role of Essential Oils in Relieving Stress

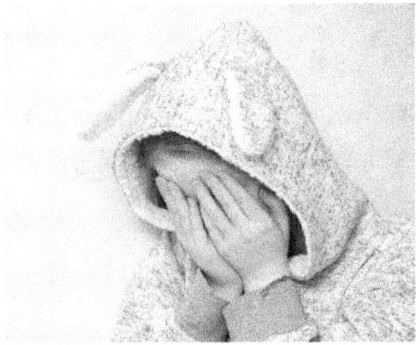

Stress can originate from different scenarios that we experience in our lives. We are lucky that there are natural techniques to support you in recovering from stress so that it will not elevate into something worse.

Thankfully, the concept of essential oils is invented because of them a lot of problems can now be cured naturally without any hassles.

They are very effective in releasing stress aside from that they can also enhance our performance and energy on everything that we do. Scientific research with essential oils particularly citrus has shown a significant improvement in their mental state.

Here are some examples of essential oil recipes that you can do at the comforts of your own home to relieve stress without undergoing any medical procedure.

Lavender and Clary Sage Blend

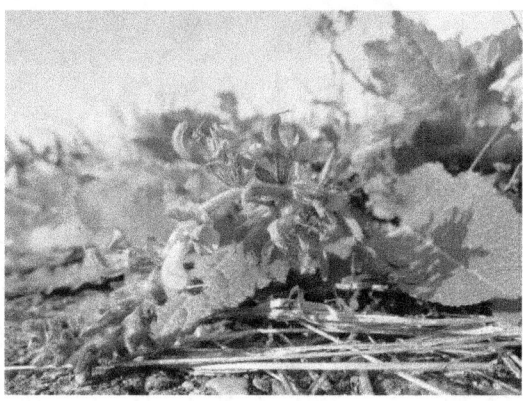

There are instances that stress can lead to sleep deprivation. The proceeding combinations of essential oils will aid you in sleeping rapidly which will result in lessening of stress in your life.

Lemon oil (5 drops)

Clary Sage (8 drops)

Lavender oil (5 drops)

Almond oil (2 drops)

Massage the combination of those essential oils among your hands and breathe in the aroma. Then continue doing it at the back of your neck and downwards. You can sense the pressure being released out of your body.

Sandal Wood Essential Oil Blend Recipe

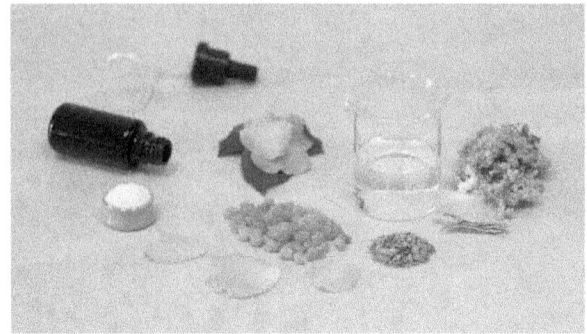

Put 5 drops of vetiver and 5 drops of sandalwood to the water that you will be used in taking a bath and then unwind while gasping the aroma.

Ylang-Ylang and Valerian Essential Oil Blend Recipe

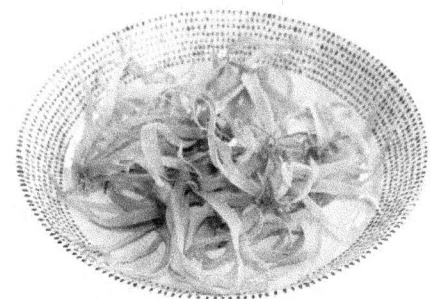

Mix 3 drops of valerian essential oil with 5 drops of ylang-ylang. Put it to you're the water that you will be using when you are going to take a bath.

Lavender and Peppermint Essential Oil Blend Recipe

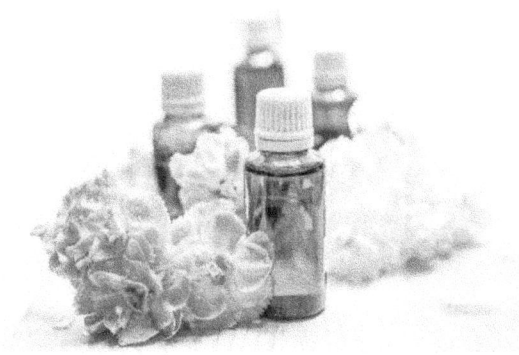

Mix 5 drops of lavender with 3 drops of peppermint essential oil or place it in a diffuser or water that you use when taking a bath.

Lavender and Chamomile Essential Oil Blend Recipe

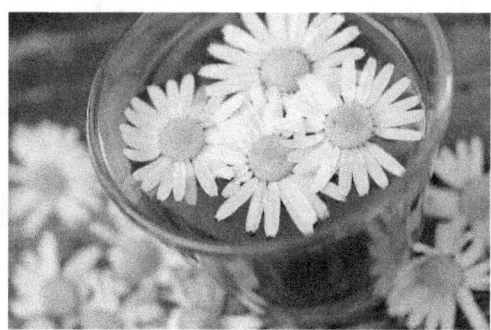

This recipe is good for any kinds of stress just mix 5 drops of lavender essential oil with 4 drops of chamomile oil. Just inhale it whenever you want to or put it on the water that you use in taking a bath.

Essential Oil Blend Recipes for Anxiety

Mix the succeeding essential oils:

Chamomile (16 drops)

Bergamot (2 drops)

Lavender (7 drops)

Geranium (7 drops)

Citrus (8 drops)

How to do it?

Place 2 tbsp of course sea salt in a container.

Place the blends inside it.

Blend them completely and cover it afterward.

Inhale this recipe three times up to 6 times a day to help you resolve your migraine problems.

Chapter 2 – Essential Oil Recipes for Relaxation

There are times when we feel that we are exhausted from the everyday work that we do because of that our energies are drained throughout our body. This is the primary reasons why we look for ways on how to rejuvenate ourselves to bring back the energy loss from the tasks that we do. One way is through the use of essential oils because it is all natural and very effective on its purpose.

Throughout the years a lot of essential oil blend recipes are created to help us relax and soothe our minds for us to function much better whenever needed. Here are some of the recipes that you can make at the comforts of your own home.

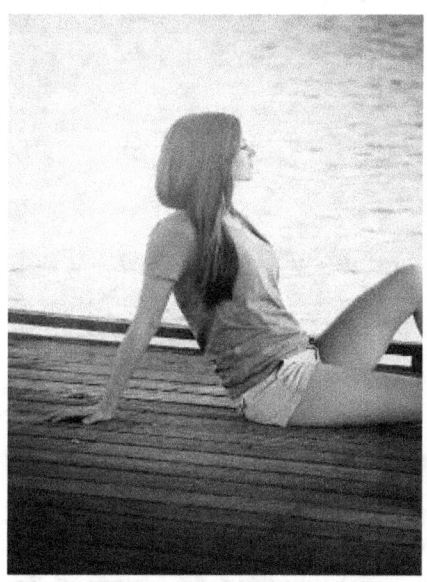

Lavender and Chamomile Blend

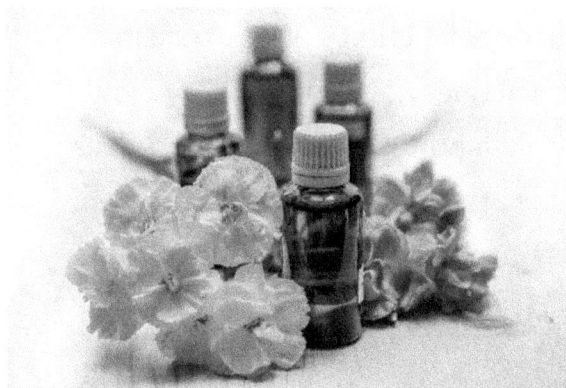

Lavender is popular among the most mainstream and flexible essential oils because it has fragrant healing benefits that can improve your general wellbeing. Since it is it can be used to beautify our skin, heal certain diseases, and restore our health.

What's more? it is also good for the development and maintenance of our brain. Lavender effects the mind similar to what medicines do. When you blend it with chamomile - another essential oil that quiets the nerves - the unwinding boosting properties are much tougher. Chamomile has been demonstrated to battle nervousness and wretchedness.

Lavender and Bergamot

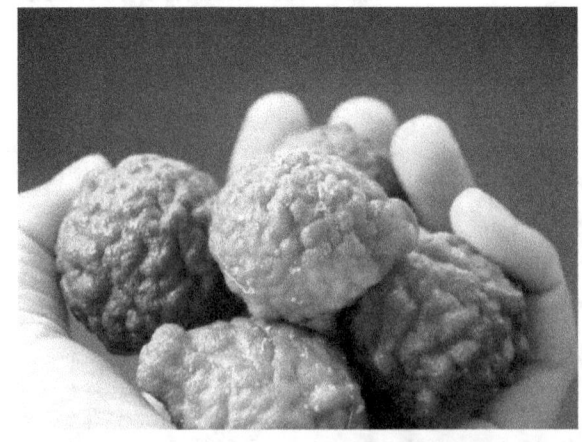

In the event that you are attempting to loosen up because of an unpleasant day, you need fragrant healing that will bring you back on track. In the event that you already have some lavender, add bergamot to add more zen to the recipe. Studies show different fragrance based treatment benefits; bergamot catches the enormous three for advancing mental unwinding, lessening your circulatory strain, pulse, and feeling of anxiety. It likewise mitigates physical agony that can meddle with genuine feelings of serenity.

Lavender, Bergamot, Frankincense, and Cedarwood

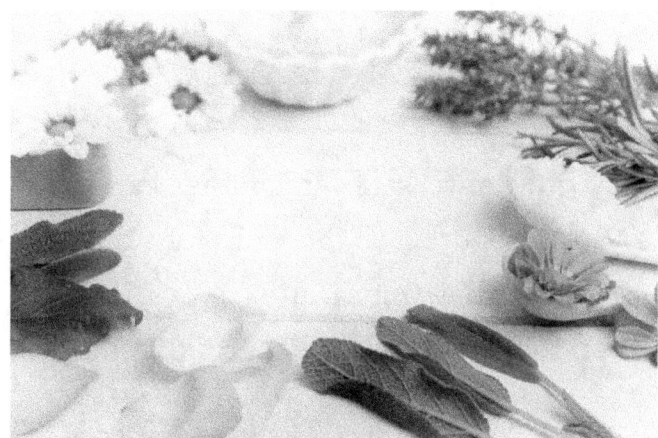

Its been logically demonstrated that, with fragrance-based treatment, you don't need to compromise your magnificence rest. As indicated by different medical professionals, an amazing tranquilizer includes blending bergamot, lavender, frankincense, and cedarwood in a jug. You can even test these oils independently to check whether they help balance your sleep deprivation.

Lemon and Eucalyptus

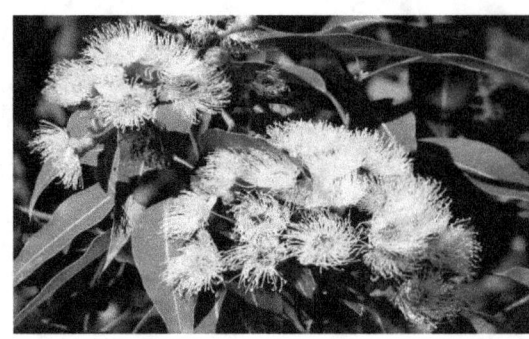

The failure to unwind can prompt interminable pressure and unstable overall health. Fortunately, the blend of lemon and eucalyptus can help mitigate your cold and sinus disease. Lemon is a phenomenal decongestant with antiviral properties, while eucalyptus encourages breathing through a stuffy nose.

Steaming your face with a towel set over your head and bowl of boiling water is unwinding in itself. Include a couple of drops of these oils for a quieting knowledge that will soothe a lot of your dilemmas regarding your health.

Frankincense, Cedarwood, and Chamomile

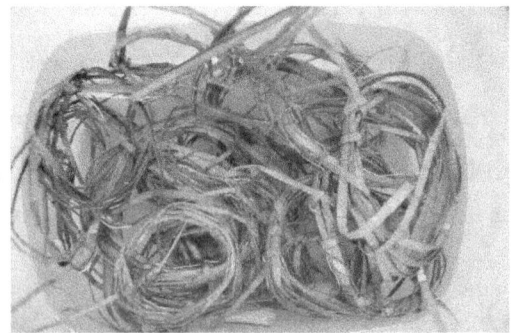

When you can't release it, attempt frankincense. This essential oil has been utilized for a considerable length of time to help individuals ponder. At the point when matched with cedarwood and chamomile, it is significantly increasingly strong in calming the brain.

Chapter 3 – Essential Oil Recipes For Healing

Believe it or not, the best essential oils that we know today are the latest in plant-based treatments. To be reasonable, ancient people practiced various distillation strategies, however, the essential oils that were removed hundreds of years prior were really different from are accessible to us today.Nevertheless, they all contained essential oils and extremely successful at avoiding and any unforeseen sickness.

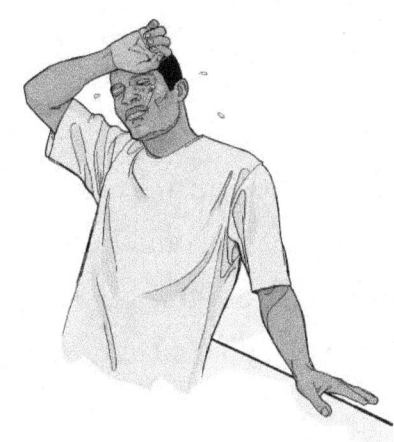

It is said that ancient people were delighted in by those in old Cyprus, Egypt and Pompeii who originally utilized herbs with refining strategies going back 3,500 B.C. This insight cruised over the Mediterranean and clearly achieved Hippocrates, who used fragrance based treatment to their immune systems a couple of hundreds of years before the happening to Christ.

As technology exchanged force to be reckoned with, the method of utilizing the best essential oils for healing from Greece went to Rome, who preferred fragrant healing and aromas.

Master the art of blending essential oils at the comforts of your own home! To help you achieve your wellbeing objectives with fundamental oils if it's not too much trouble make certain to set aside the effort to gain proficiency with the basics of aroma based treatment. The best essential oils for healing are composed of various particles that each convey various impacts on the body.

Here is the rundown of the best essential oils to use for healing

Clove (Eugenia Caryophyllata)

Clove essential oil is generally utilized as a disinfectant for infections mostly the oral ones and to wipe out a wide range of organisms to keep ailment under control. It is known to combat a lot of bacteria such as E. coli and furthermore applied significant power over Staph aureus and Pseudomonas aeruginosa which are two microscopic organisms that are the main causes of pneumonia and skin contaminations.

Eucalyptus Globulus

This essential oil is used mostly by the Aborigines for most ailments in their tribe, eucalyptus is an effective antibacterial, antispasmodic, and antiviral oil. Like clove basic oil, eucalyptus basic oil has a significant effect over Staph contaminations. Did you know that when Staph aureus comes into contact with eucalyptus oil, the dangerous bacteria have totally lost control within a span of 15 minutes!

Frankincense

This essential oil has been utilized with much success in treating issues identified with bodily functions, immune system, oral wellbeing, respiratory concerns, and stress.

Lavender

Know for its alleviating and calming properties, lavender is great for quickening the recuperating time for wounds, stings, and various type of injuries. It is loaded with cancer prevention properties. It is also assessed for its capacity to treat diabetes and anxiety in rodents.

Lemon

Different citrus fundamental oils are broadly used to have healthy nodes, to revive slow, dull skin and as a bug repellent.

Chapter 4 – Essential Oil Recipes for Sleep

Diffusing essential oils for a good rest is one of the main things that got me interested in the world of essential oils.

Like most of us, I used to wake up 1 to 2 times each night. I'd hear the pooch strolling around, or my partner would turn over, or my psyche would race with every one of the things I needed to do the following day. I just couldn't appear to get the rest I desire. I was constantly worn out the next day because I did not get the sleeping hours that I need.

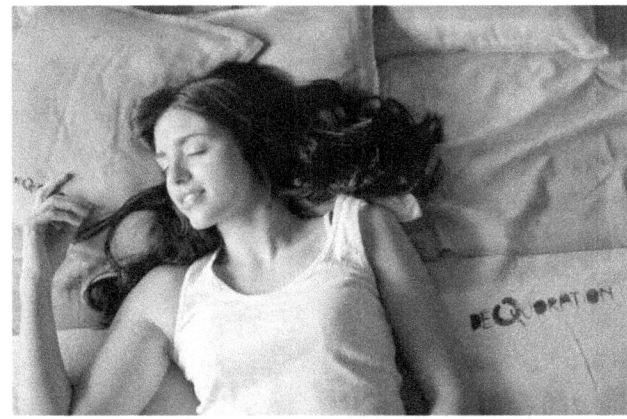

So this is when I try to experiment in using essential oils. I put 4 to 6 drops of lavender basic oil in a diffuser on the surface of my bed. Turned the diffuser on. Lie into my bed and floated off to rest.

Next thing I realized that it relieved the symptoms that I am experiencing before. I had rested straight during that time for an entire 9 hours "In any case, how could this be?" I thought it was just a coincidence.

So I attempted it again the following night. I topped off my diffuser with faucet water, and once more, I put a couple of drops of lavender essential oil in my diffuser. I transformed it on and went straight into my bed. Once more, I slept soundly as the night progressed, not awakening until I regained my consciousness back at 6:00.

There are many fundamental oils that help the psyche and body unwind My preferred essential oils that help an incredible night's rest are lavender, cedarwood, vetiver, marjoram, frankincense, bergamot, sandalwood, Roman chamomile, patchouli, and orange.

Lavender

It is generally utilized for its calming properties. It facilitates pressure and initiates unwinding.

Cedarwood

The warm and woody fragrance that is both establishing and quieting, advancing an incredible night's rest

Vetiver

This grass has a rich, fascinating smell that is really great for manipulating your moods.

Marjoram

It has a warm fragrance that quiets and lets you diminish pressure and other types of anxiousness.

Roman Chamomile

It has a sweet botanical fragrance is quieting and alleviating to the brain and body, making it a standout amongst the frequently utilized essential oils for rest

Wild Orange

It's sweet citrus fragrance and, similar to bergamot, wild orange is an adaptogen that can be empowering or calming, contingent upon what your body needs

Patchouli

The musky aroma is establishing and great for managing your feelings

Hawaiian Sandalwood

It has a rich, sweet and woody fragrance imparts quiet and unwinding. It's alleviating fragrance decreases pressure, advances enthusiastic prosperity, and has a thoughtful impact.

Recipe # 1

Lavender essential oil (2 drops)

Cedarwood essential oil (2 drops)

Recipe #2

Bergamot essential oil (4 drops)

Lavender essential oil (5 drops)

Recipe #3

Lavender essential oil (2 drops)

Wild orange essential oil (2 drops)

Recipe #4

Lavender essential oil (3 drops)

Vetiver essential oil (3 drops)

Marjoram essential oil (3 drops)

Recipe #5

Roman chamomile essential oil (4 drops)

Bergamot essential oil (3 drops)

Frankincense essential oil (3 drops)

Recipe #6

Grounding blend essential oil (4 drops)

Lavender essential oil (3 drops)

Roman chamomile essential oil (3 drops)

Recipe #7

Lavender essential oil (3 drops)

Roman chamomile essential oil (3 drops)

Marjoram essential oil (3 drops)

Recipe #8

Patchouli essential oil (3 drops)

Wild orange essential oil (2 drops)

Frankincense essential oil (3 drops)

Recipe #9

Vetiver essential oil (4 drops)

Lavender essential oil (4 drops)

Frankincense essential oil (3 drops)

Recipe #10

Lavender essential oil (4 drops)

Vetiver essential oil (4 drops)

Recipe #11

Vetiver essential oil (4 drops)

Calming blend essential oil (4 drops)

Recipe #12

3 drops patchouli essential oil

3 drops sandalwood essential oil

Chapter 5 – Essential Oil Recipes for Hair Growth

Another advantage of essential oils have is its capacity to enhance our hair. Various oils can do everything from helping the hair to sparkle and to become stronger.

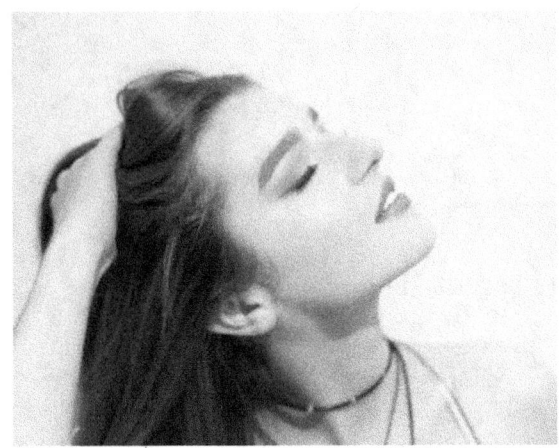

Here are the most effective essential oils for your hair:

Lavender

It can accelerate hair development. Realizing that lavender oil has properties that can create the development of cells and lessen pressure, scientists on one creature examine found that this oil had the option to produce quicker hair development in mice.

It also has antimicrobial and antibacterial properties, which can improve scalp wellbeing. Blend a few drops of lavender oil into 3 tablespoons of bearer oil, similar to olive oil or softened coconut oil, and apply it generously to your scalp. Let it sit for 10 minutes before washing it out and shampooing as you typically would. You can do this a few times each week.

Peppermint

Peppermint oil can cause a cool, shivering inclination while having a good circulation on the portion of your body that you will apply it. This can help promote the growth of new hair.

One research found that peppermint oil, when utilized on mice, expanded the number of follicles for more opportunity of growing hair. Blend 3 drops of peppermint basic oil with your preferred carrier oil. Backrub into your scalp, and let it sit for 5 minutes before washing out altogether with cleanser and conditioner.

Rosemary

If you need to improve both hair thickness and hair development, rosemary oil is a great choice because of its capacity to enhance our cells.

Blend a few drops of rosemary oil with olive or coconut oil, and apply it to your scalp. Let it sit for 10 minutes before washing it out with cleanser. Do this two times in seven days for more a desirable outcome.

Cedarwood

This essential oil is thought to promote hair development and diminish the usual male pattern baldness by adjusting the oil-producing organs in the scalp. It also has antifungal and antibacterial properties, which can treat various conditions that may add to dandruff or balding.

If you will put it into a blend with lavender, rosemary, and cedarwood it was found to diminish male pattern baldness in those with alopecia areata. Blend a couple of drops of cedarwood essential oil with 1 tbsp of carrier oil of your preference. Backrub into your scalp, and abandon it on for 10 minutes before washing it out.

Lemongrass basic oil

Dandruff can be a big problem, and having a dandruff-free scalp is a significant piece of hair wellbeing. Lemongrass oil is a very effective dandruff treatment and it is better if you will add it to your daily regimen. Blend a couple of drops into your shampoo and ensure it's rubbed really well into your scalp.

Chapter 6 – Essential Oil for Cancer and Other Diseases

I stand that one of the most useful types of herbal medicines in the world is essential oils. From triggering tranquility to calming our skin, aids healing and the combat certain illnesses, essential oils gives boundless opportunities to your well-being. I'll just clarify that the utilization of these oils is not just a trend. Essential oils have been used already by our ancestors from the different portions of the world in ancient times.

Nowadays, my family and I utilized these oils in various uses in our everyday life. The purpose of these healing objects is pretty tremendous. I'll put a rundown of it, but some ways we usually utilize essential oils comprise as medicines, for hygiene, detoxification, and etc.Why do we consider all of us must imitate us in utilizing essential oils as a basic necessity.

It's basic. We chose to utilize nonhazardous natural ways that have proven credibility in terms of their advantages, over a complete reliance on the prescribed medicines that are known for their side-effects.

Similarly, we opt to utilize own hygienic items and cleansers that are a great option because you are getting the cleansing power without the harmful chemicals. We get similar or even better outcomes while diminishing the hazards in our very own health.

I often questioned about the essential oils we prefer using to improve our overall health and prevent the formation of cancers, and also how we utilize them. This is the primary reason why I will share it to you so that you can also improve your health just like me and my family with the use of these essential oils.

Frankincense

Frankincense likely could be my absolute favorite essential oil because it fights certain tumors. It is mitigating, for one, which is imperative in the journey to recuperate from a lot of illnesses not only cancer. In particular, frankincense has been appeared to be an intense inhibitor of 5-lipoxygenase, a catalyst in charge of the immune system in the body.

It also helps support resistant capacity and anticipates sickness by duplicating white platelets and balancing invulnerable responses. It additionally improves flow, and decrease the pressure in our body. Oil of frankincense has appeared to contract and tone tissues, which speeds recovery.

Frankincense also appeared to give neurological help, including the capacity to get rid of poisons that may prompt neurological harm.

Nonetheless, it has a few advantages with regards to malignant tumor treatments, including relieving joint inflammation, equalizing hormones, empowering skin wellbeing, and helping assimilation.

Lavender

It has the phytochemicals perillyl liquor and linalool that are proven to drive malignant tumors away from our body.

It minimizes stress and supports the capacity of the immune system to perform better. Sleeping patterns are also improved with the use of this oil. Sadness and nervousness are completely taken away from our senses too. These go towards supporting the immune system in the battling of different illnesses.

Medical research has concluded that lavender essential oil is great in fighting different kinds of bacteria making the people who are using it really healthy.

Myrrh

Myrrh is considered as a very useful essential oil in the world of herbal medicines because it has a lot of incredible healing properties that. As far as disease healing is concerned, myrrh essential oil shows outstanding results in fighting malignant tumors.

It is also known to provide equilibrium in the hormones inside our body, which can be very crucial in healing. Like lavender and frankincense, It is also been utilized as a stress reliever.

Peppermint

It is a miracle oil with a wide scope of advantages. This essential oil's advantages in fighting cancers originate from its phytochemicals limonene, phytochemicals beta-caryophyllene, and beta-pinene, which are known for their effective detoxification properties.

Research says that this essential oil has the capacity to provide cell reinforcement and cancer-fighting agent properties which mostly concentrates on the prevention of tumor growth. It also contains antiangiogenic properties, which keep tumors from building up their own blood supply.

It also has antibacterial properties that make it really advantageous for fighting respiratory infection.

Turmeric

This essential oil has shown that if it is in a concentrated form, is known to battle malignant cells while advancing apoptosis resulting in a cancer-free body.

This very efficient essential oil has different advantages also that includes controlling glucose, help wounds heal rapidly, avert Alzheimer's illness, support you in getting a fit body, and simplicity joint pain.

How to Use Essential Oils for Healing?

Essential oils are so indispensable to my family's life, it's difficult to list each way we are using them! Whatever it may be, here are some top tips for utilizing essential oils in your everyday life.

- Put a drop behind your ears

  On a daily basis, I put myrrh and frankincense behind my ears and on the lymph hubs as a prophylactic (precaution insurance). Lavender or peppermint would be useful for respiratory issues, or basically to unwind. You can rub on the back of the skull, the bosoms, or the bottoms of your feet.

- Use a cool diffuser

  We want to diffuse essential oils all through our home. We do it for included mental lucidity. My office is constantly loaded up with the restorative smells of an assortment of essential oils.

- Massage into the skin

  Some basic oils, similar to peppermint and clove, are exceptionally solid and it will become perfect if you will combine it with other types of oil

- You can utilize a decent quality, natural (ideally cool squeezed) oil like coconut, olive, or jojoba to blend in a couple of drops of your preferred fundamental oil.

  You would then be able to knead this straightforward "body margarine" onto your skin. For somewhat fancier body margarine, utilize a blender to whip strong coconut oil with fundamental oil. Utilize this blend to apply straightforwardly to influenced zones, (for example, with agony, joint pain, or stomach related problems), and for a snappy mind and other medical advantages.

- Ingest Internally

  One of my top pick, because I usually combine essential oils with my soothing beverages what I usually make is a so-called "Peppermint Lemonade."

I basically take 5-10 drops of peppermint essential oil, around twelve drops of lemon (or orange or tangerine oils, contingent upon my temperament), include water, some natural green stevia, and ice in an expansive pitcher. It's a super-quick, solid refreshment that I cherish. It's likewise delectable as a hot drink (utilize hot water and exclude the ice). In case you're simply making one glass at any given moment, utilize just 1 drop of peppermint + 1 drop of citrus oil. You can likewise utilize a couple of drops of essential oils in an unfilled gel container and swallow it.

- Toothpaste

You can make an assortment of individual items utilizing natural essential oils and other non-poisonous substances such as creams, face washes, mouthwash, cleansers. A toothpaste is anything but difficult to make but it proved me wrong because with the use of natural frankincense, myrrh, and coconut oil it became as easy as 1, 2, and 3.

Conclusion

That was a long ride, I hope that you have learned a lot from the essential oil recipes that we have tackled a while ago. Just one piece of advice before we part ways, I suggest that you must be creative when it comes to blending the various essential oils. The primary reason for this is that the recipes of essential oil blends are not just limited to the ones that are listed here because you can actually make one of your own depends on your needs.

Just make sure to study the different oils that are in this book so that the next time you plan to make your own recipe you will know the use of each essential oil which will help you make a very astounding recipe in the future. But before anything else I would like to discuss to you the key points that you should remember if you want to use essential oils.

Quality

This is important to the point that it bears rehashing. Continuously utilize a top-quality, therapeutic essential oil. It ought to be ensured natural, and 100% unadulterated. Check the notoriety of your provider, and guarantee there are no fillers or added substances.

Keep oils from delicate territories

Essential oils are nature's powerhouses. Remember they are 40-50 times stronger than the plant itself. A few oils are progressively "fiery" than others. Some taste superior to other people.

Oregano is one that can consume a bit when you ingest it legitimately. Peppermint requires alert, and generally does best with a transporter oil when applying to the skin. Never apply essential oils to touchy territories of the body, including the private areas or close to your eyes.

You ought to likewise test new oils to guarantee there are no responses before applying too generously.

You can begin by completing a sniff trial of the oil in the jug. In an instance that appears to be fine, at that point apply a spot of oil to within your wrist or arm, include a drop of oil and hold on to check whether there is any redness, tingling, or swelling. Everyone's body is unique so you may need to attempt various oils to see which ones feel best to you.

Do not heat up oils

You've most likely observed or even have one of those oil burners for utilizing essential oils. What you can be sure of is that warming these oils decimates their healing properties. It's in every case best to utilize a cool diffuser. These are abundant and monetarily evaluated on the web.

Keep out of Children

Continuously be mindful when utilizing essential oils with kids. Dispersion is the most secure. For direct application, it's critical to weakening the more grounded oils, particularly with a decent oil. When making body spreads or back rub oils for kids, utilize 1 drop of essential oil to 4 tablespoons of other oils.

This will weaken the essential oil enough to make it progressively in the middle of the road and more secure for your kid. Be mindful so as not to put close to the eyes and dependably complete an allergy test first.

One word is very important in creating your own essential oil recipe which is "creativity" always apply that when you plan to make a recipe. So that's it I wish you good luck to your future endeavors.

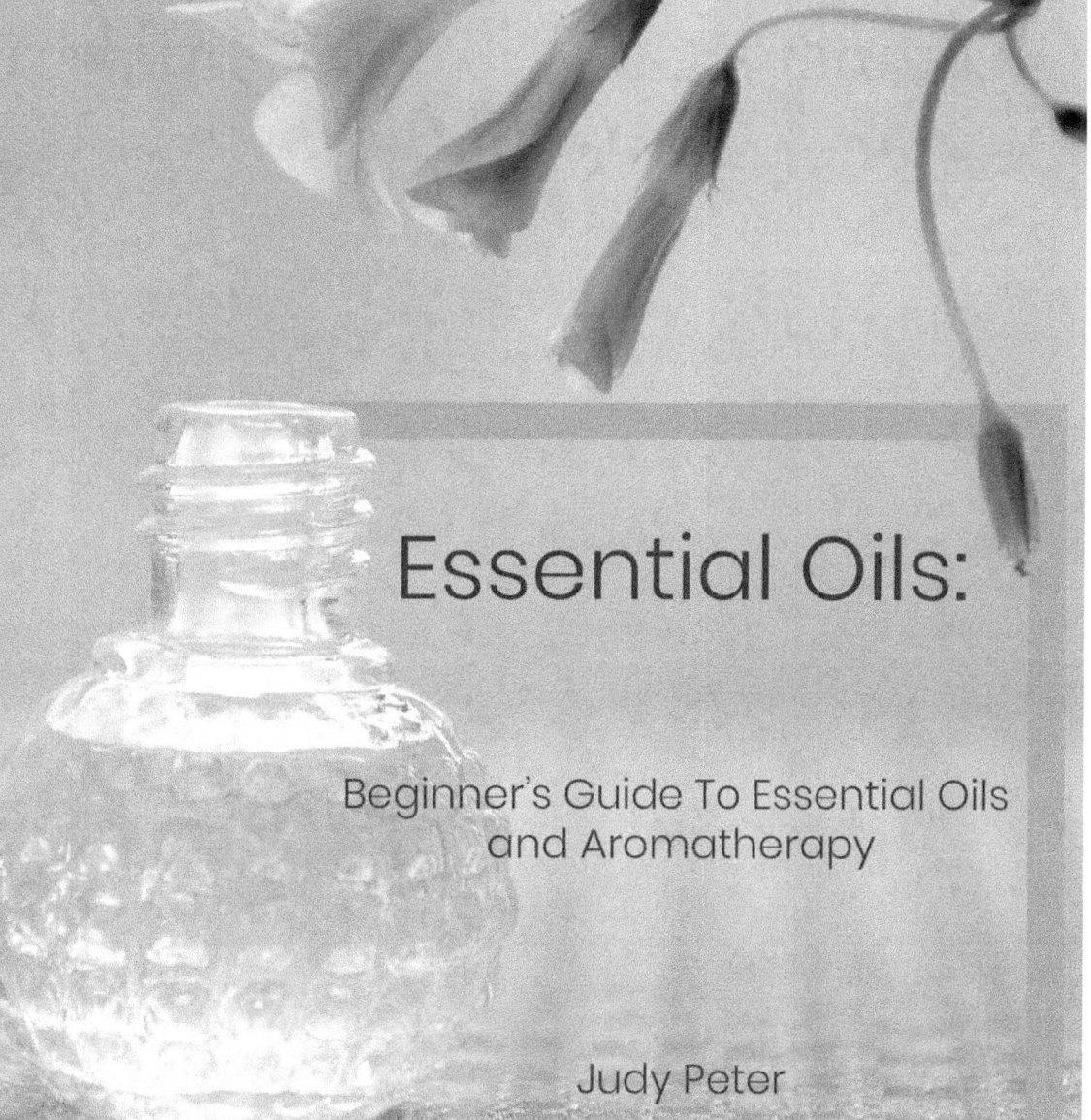

Essential Oils:

Beginner's Guide To Essential Oils and Aromatherapy

Judy Peter

Essential Oils:
Beginner's Guide To Essential Oils and Aromatherapy

Introduction: The Soothing Satisfaction of Essential Oil

Essential oils are essentially just a much more concentrated batch of plant oils already found in nature. Lemon essential oil for example, is simply the natural oil extracted from a lemon in a much more powerfully condensed form. This oil is usually created by way of distillation—produced through hot steam. This method makes sure that the most potent batch of oil is created with the least amount of effort.

The main essence of the oils once extracted are usually paired with a base or "carrier" oil and then further refined for human consumption. If your oil is not mixed with a carrier agent, caution must be exercised as some essential oils have been known to be so powerful that they cause irritation to exposed skin.

It is for this reason that diluting just a few drops in a carrier oil are usually recommended. People have come to greatly benefit from the use of specific essential oils whether by simply inhaling them through aromatherapy or rubbing them directly into the skin during a massage.

Aromatherapy in particular has shown much promise when it comes to improving mood and other mental conditions. Our nose as it turns out is very much connected to our emotions—the nose actually links right up to glands in our limbic system such as the hippocampus which is a major center for both our emotions and our all too often limited—attention spans. By simply inhaling certain chemical compounds our moods can be lifted and concentration can be improved.

The practice of aromatherapy through the use of essential oils has been used for thousands of years. It is for this reason that many ancient religions use incense during their religious services because the sweet aroma of the incense is often viewed as necessary for bringing the congregants into just the right mental state. Those who participated in these time-honored rituals knew just how fulfilling they were. But you don't have to wait until the next mass to benefit from aromatherapy.

This book provides you with detailed recipes of essential oils that you can put together in your own home. So, get ready. Because now you too are about to discover the soothing satisfaction that these essential oils can offer.

Chapter 1: How Aromatherapy Works

The nose of course is the organ that fosters our sense of smell but it runs much deeper than that. The nose is actually a bit of a messenger for the other important systems of our body, playing a major role in our daily function. So, having that said, before we delve into our aromatherapy recipes, let's take a brief look on just how it is that the nose works.

Basic Function of the Nose

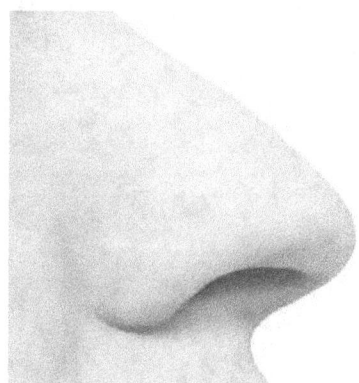

The nose is part of a complicated sensory system in our body which stand on the front line to sort out all of the chemical compounds that we are bombarded with on a daily basis. Whether those compounds are molecules rising up from a freshly cooked steak, or the smell of your car's smoking radiator.

Our nose alerts us ahead of time to what we are about to get into. The nose is important as an information system, informing us of what we are up against. But it does more than alert us to smelly things nearby, it also processes those same chemical compounds that we inhale, taking specific smell molecules and combining them to receptors that influence our mood, memory, and emotion. You see, our nose plays a much bigger role than most of us care to realize.

Despite alerting us to strong odors and fragrances, the nose is constantly working on even the most subconscious of levels influencing our mood and temperament. Just about everywhere we go we encounter miniscule little smell molecules are wafting up our nostrils. After passing into our nostrils, they dock with special chemical sensory receptors and impart some very specific information to your body as well as providing the receptors with a very specific stimulus.

That stimulus could be for energy, to go to sleep, or even to raise the metabolism –all depending on what the chemical compound has to impart upon these nasal receptors. And just think about it, all of these complex exchanges occur faster than you can smell the afternoon popcorn! This is just the basic function of our nose at work.

Application Methods

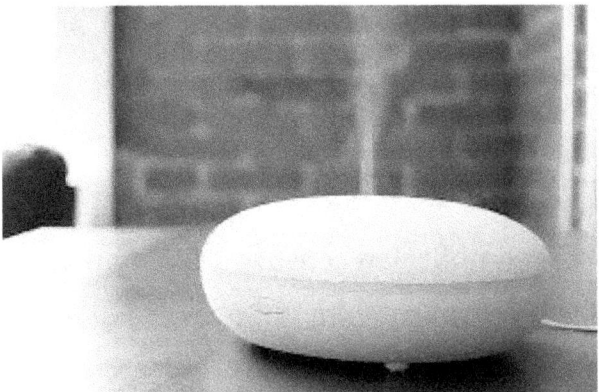

Now that we know how the nose works, let's look at some application methods for aromatherapy. The most basic way to use essential oils for aromatherapy would be just to inhale their scent right out of the bottle. I personally have done this myself to treat my asthma with a variety of essential oils I keep around, such as peppermint and frankincense.

In those moments that I feel tightness in my chest and receive the distinct indication of a bad episode of asthma coming on, I just pull out one of the bottles take the lid off and breathe in as deep as I possibly can

For a quick fix, this method of application is helpful. And without any extra equipment or elaborate preparation, benefits can be gleaned. But although useful, this method leaves much to be desired. For a more powerful effect, you could simply deposit a few drops of the oil in a container of boiling or near boiling water. This water can be heated up either through the use of a tea kettle or simply by placing a container filled with water into the microwave and heating it up for a few minutes on high.

However, it is that you do it, as soon as the oil hits the hot water it will rise up as steam. Once the steam starts to flow, simply lean over the container and breathe in the aroma. The most effective way of using these oils in aromatherapy however would be to actually purchase and use a diffuser. The diffuser is an appliance that mechanically spreads the aroma of essential oils through the air through steam. This is the basic gist of how aromatherapy works.

Chapter 2: Aromatic Anxiety Relief Recipes

Anxiety is a big problem in the modern world. We are all busy and rushing from one place to the next. Not only that, even in our free time most of us tend to be constantly looking at a screen—whether its our laptop, tablet or phone, we are constantly fiddling with a technological device in order to keep up. But all of this constant stimulation is causing our brains to go into hyperdrive.

So much so in fact, that the next time you are forced to look away from your phone and do absolutely nothing, the adjustment can be downright painful. Simply having to stare up at a red traffic light for example, and you find yourself becoming increasingly anxious for that said light to turn green. The mind that is used to constantly running is now forced to sit still with nothing to do, and it doesn't like it!

Having trouble putting your overworked mind into standby mode for mundane tasks is an indication that things are getting out of whack. It is a clear sign of an overloaded system in need of some pure and simple anxiety relief! The recipes presented in this chapter are geared to help you breathe out that stress, worry and anxiety and breathe in the aroma of calm and soothing essential oils.

Rose Essential Oil

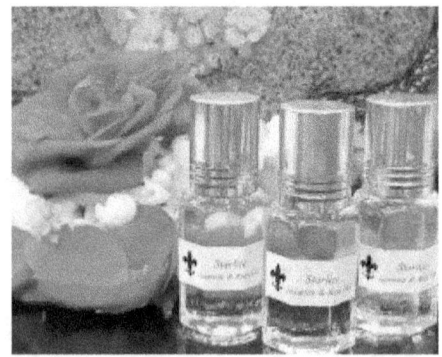

Rose essential oil comes directly from fresh cut roses. If anyone has ever asked you to slow down to "stop and smell the roses", it's because the scent of this flower is able to put people at ease simply by smelling it.

It is for this reason that essential rose oil, which is basically just a much more highly concentrated batch of that same aroma from a fresh cut rose, is so effective at lessoning the symptoms that result from of an anxious and overworked mind. Rose essential oil is so powerful in fact, that routine regimens of it has been shown to actually calm the heart and reduce the incidence of high blood pressure in the body.

If you need a natural way to calm your racing heart and mind, this oil could be just what you are looking for. It opens airways, slows the pulse and alleviates any lingering brain fog from the mind. In order to create your own batch of essential rose oil for aromatherapy, just add a few drops of rose oil to your choice of carrier oil and burn it as incense or run it through a good diffuser.

Allow yourself to then gradually inhale the aroma for a few hours and you will be feeling great. Yes, it truly is a good thing when we to take some time to smell the roses! Try this blend of rose essential oil today!

Geranium Essential Oil

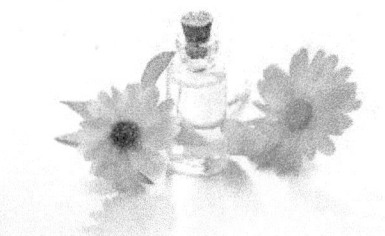

The Geranium flower is great when it comes to relieving anxiety. Geranium oil is actually very similar to rose oil in composition but for those that are interested—geranium oil is usually a whole heck of a lot cheaper than rose oil. So, having that said, for a cheaper yet still highly effective anxiety reliever this essential oil could be your go-to source.

Geranium oil is indeed an essential ingredient. This oil produces a very nice scent that fills the room with a gentle almost citrus-like aroma. Just place 4 or 5 drops into a good carrier oil, and toss it into an incense burner or proper diffuser, and you are good to go. Give yourself 30 to 40 minutes to breathe in the aroma that is produced. For an extra boost you could also add 2 drops of clary sage oil. Just breathe in the aroma until you feel yourself begin relax!

Bergamot and Lavender Essential Oil Mix

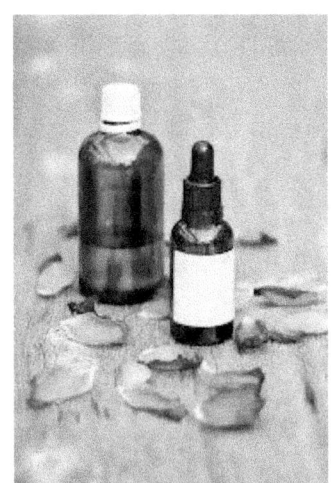

The reason why both Bergamot and Lavender are crucial ingredients when it comes to relieving anxiety is due to a little something called "linalyl acetate". This chemical has been shown to relax both the body and the mind as soon as our nose encounters it.

This combination of bergamot and lavender also provides us with a rather distinctive and pleasing aroma as well. Just add a couple drops of Bergamot along with at least one drop of lavender into a proper carrier oil, distribute to an incense burner, and allow the sweet scent to fill the room. The feeling is almost immediate, and you will be feeling better in no time. Go ahead and give it try!

Neroli Essential Oil

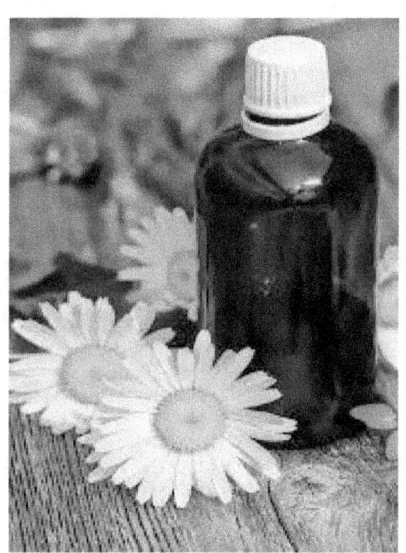

Neroli essential oil is a true workhouse when it comes to essential oils. This powerful and refreshing essential oil has been known to actually slow down the quickened pulse, and bring clarity to the troubled mind.

This calming and classy oil refreshes the entire system simply from breathing in its aroma. Neroli originates from the Seville orange tree. It is actually the orange peels from which neroli oil is extracted. The name is said to have its origins in the Italian town of Nerola where this essential oil was widely manufactured and used by the locals.

This essential oil was used in religious ceremonies as incense as well as by those simply wishing to take the edge off of their own edginess. And don't just take my word for it—take the word of science. Because this oil has been shown in several scientific studies to the improve moods of those who partake of it.

One of the most recent in fact had a group of women dealing with depression and anxiety breathe in neroli as a form of aromatherapy while another group of women breathed in just basic almond oil. Without being told which type of oil they were breathing, time and time again, the group of women who inhaled neroli saw a relief of their symptoms. Whereas the women who partook of just basic almond oil so no difference.

This study clearly indicates a connection between neroli and the alleviation of anxiety. In order to start your own aromatherapy regimen with neroli, simply add 4 or 5 drops to a carrier oil and inhale as incense, or place a few drops with a cup of water into your diffuser. You will feel a lot better for it!

Frankincense Essential Oil

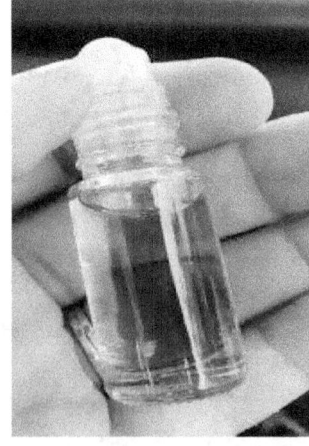

Hailing from the African continent, this ancient essential oil has been held as a prized possession the world over, for literally thousands of years. And for good reason. The rare chemicals within this essential oil have the ability to relieve stress and bring back mental clarity like no other. Just about anyone feeling down in the dumps will feel remarkably better once the fragrance of frankincense has been introduced.

It is for this reason that religions all over the globe have burned incense of frankincense during religious ceremonies. And if you can recall your Christmas nativity, frankincense and myrrh played quite a pivotal role there as well. Frankincense in some places was actually valued to be worth more than gold. Demonstrating that the ancients placed just as much worth on having proper mental clarity as we do today.

Because the aroma of this oil has quite a way of easing away stress and bringing the mind to a proper state of balance. So. without further ado, let's get started on your own batch of frankincense. Just add a few drops to a good base, carrier oil, place inside your incense burner or diffuser and allow the aroma to gradually release in a centralized part of your home. Now get ready to breathe in the majestic relaxation that only this powerful and potent essential oil can bring about.

Cypress Essential Oil

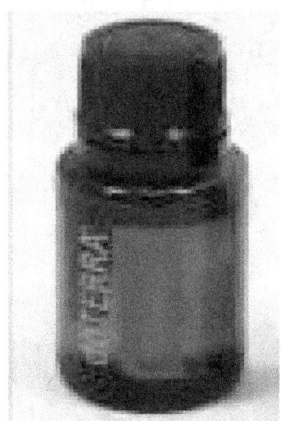

Coming from the cypress tree—this essential oil has long been prized for its ability to reduce the stress in those that come to use it. The oil itself is extracted through a process of steam distillation aimed at the tree's branches and needles.

The oil has a powerful sedative like quality that creates a great feeling of relaxation without making you drowsy. But the aroma of this oil not only calms you down it also puts you at ease with a truly content feeling. The best way to use cypress essential oil is to mix 5 drops of it with a cup of hot water and pour it right into your diffuser

You could also simply add the mix to a hot bath if you would prefer. Just give it about an hour or so to work and soon you will be feeling relaxed and at peace. If you are indeed suffering from stress and anxiety the essential oil recipes presented in this chapter are a great resource for you to have on hand.

Chapter 3: Essential Oil Recipes for Energy and Focus

In the non-stop world of today it seems that we are staying up later and setting our alarm clocks back earlier, and yet we are still never quite seeming to find the time or energy needed to stay on task. Our minds aimlessly wander and we find ourselves missing deadlines as we get stuck in the drift.

For most the go-to solution for this problem would be a good cup of coffee but too much coffee can take its physiological toll, leading to sleeplessness, irritability and anxiety. Is there a healthier alternative? Look no farther than the soothing scent of essential oils! Many of us could use a little mental boost when it comes to our energy and focus—here in this chapter we will show you how to do just that!

<u>Lemon Essential Oil</u>

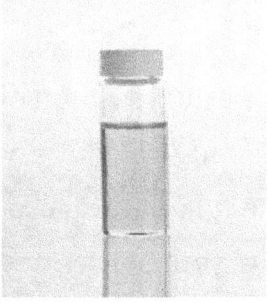

Lemons are one of nature's wonder fruits. Lemons are good for a wide variety of purposes and when condensed down into an essential oil their attributes become even more pronounced. Lemon essential oil as soon as it is inhaled works to relax both breathing and blood vessels, slowing down the heart rate and bringing about a natural sense of calm and contentment.

If you are feeling stressed out and could use a little boost, you really need to give this recipe a try. It's quick, it's painless, and most importantly—it's effective! The ingredients are quite simple, just add anywhere between 5 to 7 drops of lemon essential oil into a good incense burner or diffuser and breath in the resulting steam over the next few hours. It's a weekend getaway without ever leaving the house!

Peppermint and Cinnamon Essential Oil Mix

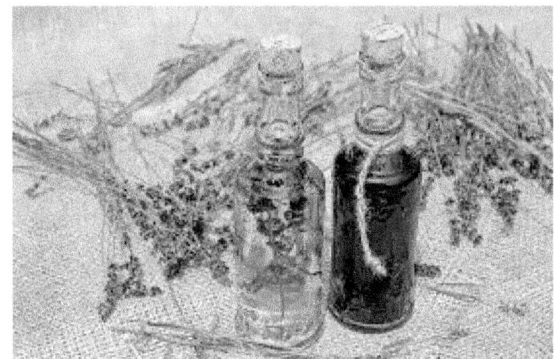

Peppermint is yet another powerful essential oil that serves a wide variety of purposes yet in particular, this oil has been found to be quite a bit of use in the form of an energy booster. If you have ever breathed in the full, natural aroma of peppermint you can probably attest to the fact that it tends to draw in your senses.

Cinnamon complements peppermint and enhances its powerful draw. Keeping that in mind, here is a special blend just for you. In order to create this mix, you will need to add 5 drops of peppermint oil and 4 drops of cinnamon oil to a carrier oil. Once mixed together, you can burn as incense or in your diffuser. Breathe in deep because the effects are almost immediate.

Rosemary Essential Oil

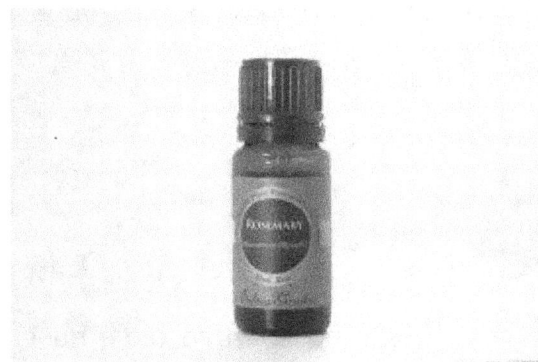

Rosemary is a great stress buster and also helps to improve our concentration and focus. A regular regimen of this essential oil helps us to make the best of our day as our increased attention span gets to work. You will find that incessant worry slipping away as you focus on the most immediate task at hand. And its powerful! Just a few drops of this stuff will do you! Add just 3 or 4 drops of this oil to a carrier base, place into your incense burner or diffuser and you are ready to roll!

The aroma produced has a pleasant, woodsy kind of feel to it. Think of that refreshing feeling when you step onto a forest trail in a nature park and you will have an idea of the pleasing aroma that rosemary essential oil can produce.

Eucalyptus Essential Oil

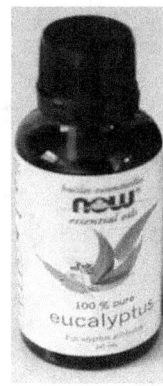

Eucalyptus provides what has been described as a cool and refreshing aroma. The act of breathing in this oil provides us with an energetic boost that resets and reboots our entire system. The chemical compounds released bond directly with special receptors in the nose and get to work.

Inhalation of the fumes produced by this essential oil has also been known to reduce the onset of headaches as well as relieve congested sinuses, making it an excellent choice for allergy sufferers.

As it turns out, Eucalyptus essential oil also doubles as an antibacterial agent and by burning it in a room, the resulting residue works to clear out any pesky bacteria that may be present, including dangerous hard to reach molds. So, as well as keeping you alert and focused, this essential oil also keeps your home and health in pretty good shape as well.

In order to create your own batch of eucalyptus essential oil just add about 6 drops of eucalyptus oil to a ½ a cup of water mixed with 2 tablespoons of cornstarch. Mix these ingredients together well and add to an incense burner or diffuser. Allow the aroma to fill the room you are in and breathe in the aroma. Eucalyptus is quite a refreshing blend that will have you back for more!

Lime Essential Oil

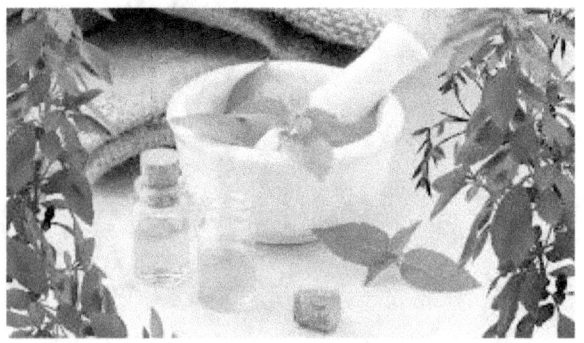

Lime essential oil is good by itself or combined with the aforementioned lemon essential oil. Lime just like lemon is good at uplifting mood and boosting general energy levels of those who use it. It has a very clean scent and can be used just about anywhere. Be warned however that lime does tend to have a rather powerful aroma and having that said not everyone likes the smell of lime.

This is more a demonstration of personal preference than anything else however, and if the aroma is pleasing to you, it does indeed do well to waken up the senses. In order to give yourself your own dose of lime essential oil, simply place a few drops of lime oil along with ½ a cup of water into a diffuser and give yourself at least an hour to slowly breath in the aroma as it diffuses out into the surrounding environment.

Pine Essential Oil

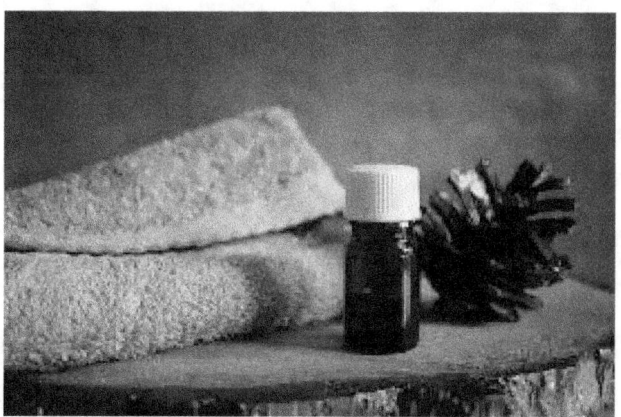

As pure as a pine tree—pine essential oil provides a pristine blend of energy enhancing aroma! This essential oil can be mixed with cedar for extra effect or just used as is. Take 4 or 5 drops and place them in your diffuser along with a good carrier oil and breath in deep! After the first 10 to 15 minutes you should be feeling alert and focused. Try some pine essential oil today!

Chapter 4: Essential Oil Recipes for Immune Health

Our health is everything. If we are not feeling at our best our work as well as our downtime will both suffer for it. And what is it that protects and guarantees our health more than anything else? The biggest vanguard of our well-being will always be our immune system.

You can think of our immune system as an invisible shield that keeps out harmful biological agents. If that wall of immunity begins to be compromised these agents will begin to break through and wreak havoc on our health. Fortunately for us, there are many essential oils that can help to boost our immune health. Keep reading to find out more about them!

Ginger Essential Oil

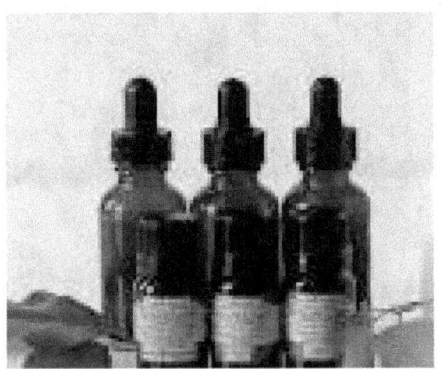

Ginger essential oil is a great immune booster. Ginger is said to have originated in China and since has spread to many other parts of the world. The oil itself is usually extracted from the root of the ginger plant. Ginger has been used for thousands of years as an additive to meals due to both its flavor and its seeming ability of aiding the stomach to digest food.

Ginger oil has many anti-inflammatory properties and these properties work well to boost a faltering immune system. Just add a few drops of ginger essential oil to a carrier oil, add a tablespoon of water and you are good to go. Place this mix into an incense burner or diffuser, sit back and inhale the resulting aroma.

Oregano Essential Oil

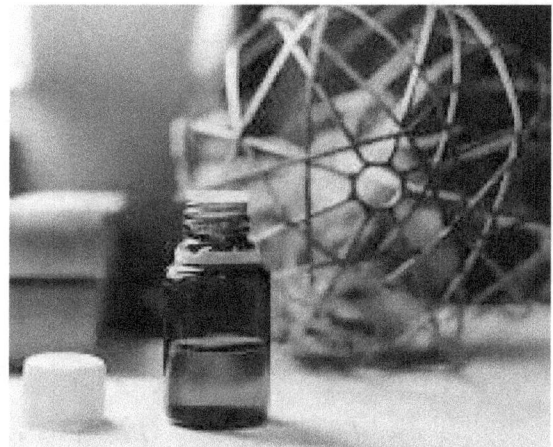

Most of us are probably primarily familiar with oregano as an ingredient in our food, but trust me, it does much more than simply enrich the flavor of our pasta! Oregano contains something called thymol and another little something called carvacrol. Both of these elements are known immune boosters.

Oregano oil comes with plenty of antioxidants that help to ensure that the body keeps a good equilibrium when it comes to keeping out harmful biological agents. Add 5 drops of oregano oil to ½ a cup of water, and mix with a carrier oil. Place inside your incense burner or diffuser. And that's it, folks!

Saffron Essential Oil

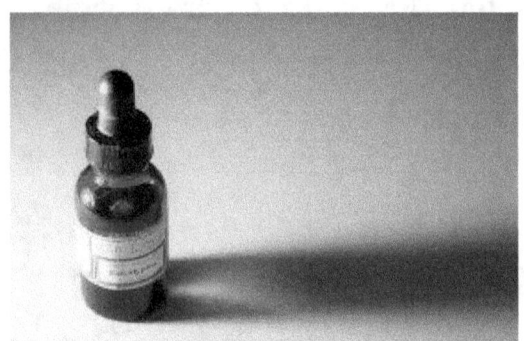

An exotic spice found in the climes of Southern Europe; saffron is one of the most sought-after herbs on the planet. Just one pound of saffron can at times cost over a thousand dollars. Not to worry however folks, because its true—just a dab of this stuff will do you! This oil is so potent that just a few drops should do the trick.

Taken from the stems of the saffron plant; the essential oil produced does wonders for the overtaxed immune system. Saffron can actually help promote a healthier cardiovascular system and boost the metabolic rate of the body which in tur supports a stronger and more robust immune system. Just put two or three drops of Saffron combined with a suitable carrier oil, into your incense burner or diffuser, and you will soon see some pretty nifty results!

Astragalus Essential Oil

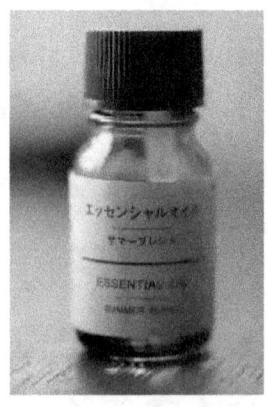

Used for countless centuries by Chinese herbalists, astragalus has been known to strengthen even the weakest of immune systems. The elderly in particular have shown much promising results through regular aromatherapy sessions with astragalus essential oil. So, just where does this immune boosting power come from?

Well—for one thing astragalus has a hefty dose of antioxidants, which are always quite good for stimulating our body's immune system. Astragalus also helps our circulation and cardio function. which in turn helps our body to keep our immune system well regulated and at its best.

So, just add one drop with a cup of water and place them into your diffuser or incense burner. Just a drop or two will do you—let your incense and diffuser do the rest!

Echinacea Essential Oil

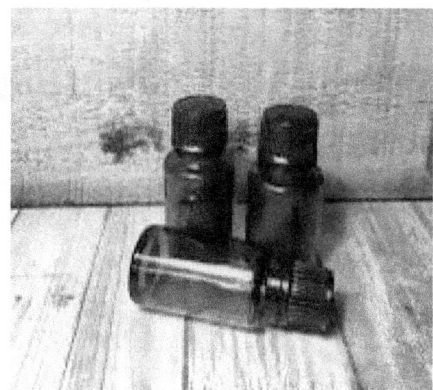

Echinacea has both antiviral and antibiotic properties and as such has been used for thousands of years the world over to aid those that are feeling a bit under the weather.

If you are sick and could use an immune boost, echinacea essential oil would be a good place for you to turn for some relief. The reason for this being that the oil from this plant contain polysaccharides.

What are polysaccharides you might ask? They are special protein building blocks needed by the body, and the reason why they are good for the immune system is due to their ability to activate white blood cells—our bodies mighty gatekeepers and defenders against biological disease.

Having that said, in order to create your own echinacea essential oil treatment, just take 4 drops of echinacea oil, 2 tablespoons of water, and mix with a good carrier oil. Add this to either an incense burner, or a diffuser, give yourself about an hour to breathe in the resulting aroma, and you are ready to go.

Cedar Essential Oil

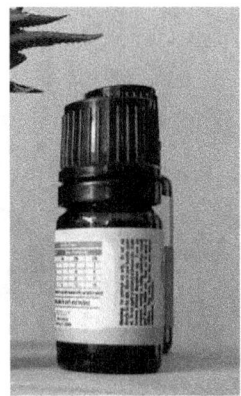

In its raw form, cedar essential oil holds much promise when it comes to boosting the immune system. This oil is obtained through direct steam distillation from pieces of cedar taken directly from a tree.

The trees that they are taken from are typically in cold or mountainous regions. Just think of the Alps and your mind is on the right track of where this oil is naturally found.

The main elements found within cedar are bedta cedrane, alpha cedrane, cedrol, widdrol, and thujopsene—all of which are known immune boosters. Their names may be hard to pronounce, but their effect is nothing short of extraordinary. So, let's get you started. For this recipe take 3 drops of cedar oil and mix it with 1 drop of cypress and 1 drop of rosemary. Add this mixture to diffuser, and allow the aroma to fill the air.

Orange Essential Oil

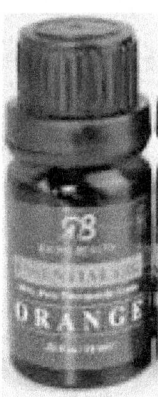

If you have ever had a cold in your life, then someone somewhere has more than likely recommended you to drink some orange juice. And there is most certainly a good reason for that since oranges are a well-known immune booster.

Orange is known to insulate the body against germs. Not only that, orange essential oil stimulates the lymphatic system. What does that mean? Well, if you have been suffering through a killer cold, it means that your nose that had previously been running like a faucet, will finally get some much-needed relief!

Orange essential oil also works as preventative medicine helping to boost your immune system enough so that you don't get that said cold in the first place! In order to create your own batch of orange essential oil to use in aromatherapy just take 3 drops of orange oil, add in one drop of jasmine oil and add to a good carrier oil such as almond, place in an incense burner or diffuser and breathe in the air!

If you are in need of a serious immune booster, give this one a try. You are going to love it! And the same could be said for all of the immune boosting oils presented here in this final chapter of this book.

Conclusion: Just a Matter of Finding the Right Ingredients

Essential oils are powerful champions of health. Several years of experience are not necessary for you to figure this out. All it really takes is a few whiffs of a strong batch of essential oil recipes and you will quickly become a believer for yourself. The natural world has indeed endowed humanity with a priceless treasure when it comes to essential oils.

In the past people believed that there was something almost sacred and supernatural in the way that these essential oils managed to get people delivered from their maladies.

But looking back at this ancient practice through a more modern lens we realize that it isn't magic that is causing this revitalization, it's a strong physiological response to just the right motivating chemicals.

This doesn't at all take away from the life changing abilities of these oils, it just helps us to better understand the ways in which they work so that we can utilize them to their fullest potential. That is the main drive and purpose of this entire book.

And I sincerely hope that the recipes presented here will be able to aid you in recovering from whatever may be troubling you. Because in the end its all just a matter of finding the right ingredients.

Thank you for reading and good luck!

Repellents:

Non-Toxic And Easy To Make Repellents
To Protect Yourself From Harmful Insects

Lester Polly

Repellents

Non-Toxic And Easy To Make Repellents To Protect Yourself From Harmful Insects

Introduction

As we all know throughout the world there are millions of species of insects present and not all of them are friendly. In fact, some of them are even deadly because they carry venomous substances on their systems. However, there are some friendly insects that we knew such as butterflies and we would love to see them fly by because they are colorful and gentle.

So what we will tackle about in this book are the insects that can bring us significant harm particularly on our health and our overall wellbeing. How did I say so? An insect bite can carry diseases such as malaria, dengue, allergies, and even HIV! Mostly, mosquitoes are the carrier of the large percentage of diseases that are brought to us by insects.

I remember before when I was still a child I was really frightened because I caught an allergy that is due to an insect bite as far as I can remember it is a bite from a bug that I got out of bed.

This is the primary reason as I grow old I am always conscious about insects and I do not want them near my skin. So I did some research on how to create my own insect repellents because the repellents that can be bought on the grocery stores and pharmacies tend to have a negative effect on my skin.

Luckily, because of hard work and research, I was able to make my first all-natural insect repellent and I was very happy. Since then I had fun making different insect repellents for various insects which became my hobby, so I decided to write it on this book to impart my knowledge to you and use it for your own advantage.

The recipes are really easy to create because there are no complex ingredients that are included in the recipes so expect that you can create them easily. Let us not delay the learning anymore by starting it off immediately with the first chapter in which I will give you some background about insects so that you can understand them.

I believe that it is a crucial matter in order to repel them away from your skin. We will start now so brace yourselves from the knowledge that you will learn throughout this eBook.

Chapter 1 – The Effects of Getting Bitten By Insects

Figuring out how to hike will give you an all-out fulfillment since it gives you that feeling of testing your sturdiness and experience the fun since you will be going to visit places with good sceneries. Along these lines, this sort of activity is somewhat hazardous because this type of activity can impose you to various issues like exposing you to a wide range of bugs.

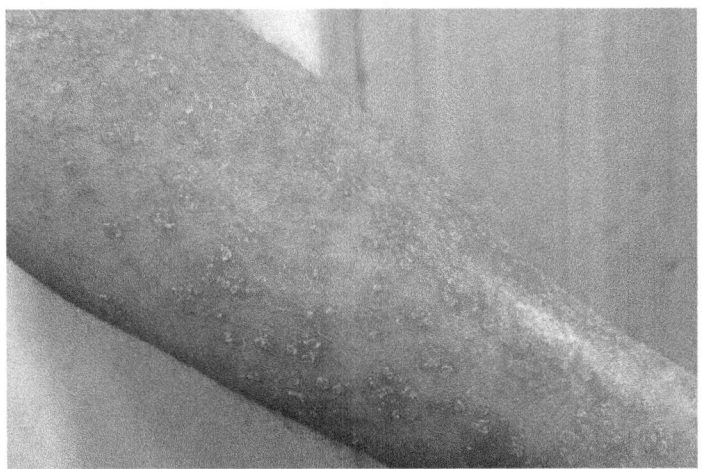

Some of them are harmless they simply love to stay nearby, while others can bring sickness that should be restored on the grounds that it can give us a destructive impact on our body Among these creepy insects are the mosquitoes, ticks, honey bees, wasps, hornets, black flies, bugs and ants, they might be delicate in the eye, however one little bite can expedite a genuine impact our wellbeing.

By being cautious and practicing effective insect counteractive action is one of the greatest things that hikers can do to avert sickness and spreading unwanted diseases. These are the common insect-cause ailments experienced by hikers, are Malaria and Japanese Encephalitis although curable it is much better for us to prevent it rather than to cure it.

Find out About Insect Behavior

Initially, know where they colonize or residing place with the goal so that you will know where to eliminate them and where the ailments transmission happened.

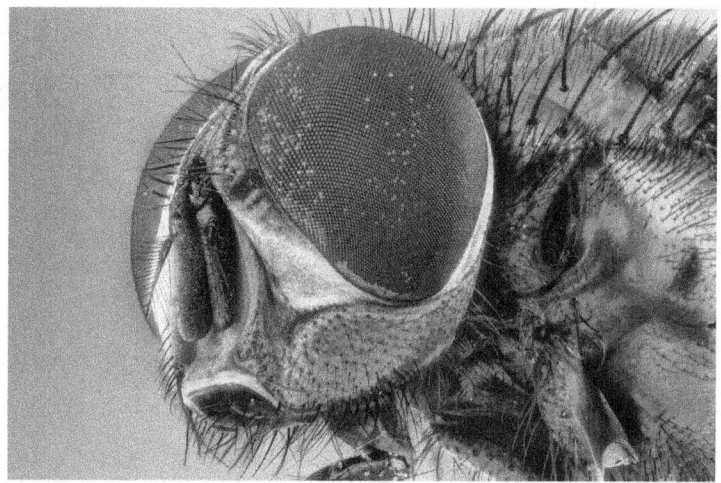

Next, find out about the insect's conduct. This will incredibly assist you with understanding whether the place that you want to travel can bring you significant exposure to those living organisms.

- What is their condition? Do they reside the inside, outside, or both?

- When would they say they are most dynamic, time? AM or PM?

- Are they present all year or do they are only seasonal?

- Do they live in urban or rustic regions?

- Are they equipped for conveying sicknesses transmitted to individuals?

Simple bite or sting?

The indications of insect bites can vary on the type of the insect and the affectability of the individual who is bitten. For instance, a few people may have little experience of irritation after they are bitten, which can go on for a minute. Others may build up an extreme resistance to it which is a good thing, however, some of us might be really affected even with one little bite which can lead to nasty swelling and even infection. Just as insects that bite harmlessly painful or not and the worst thing is you'll encounter an insect that has venom on them.

The insects that sting include:

- *bees (bumble bees and honey bees)*

- *wasps*

- *hornets*

These stinging insects are dynamic and appear on the mid part of summer to the latter part of it when the workers search for foods to provide to their rulers that they can use for the winter season.

Here are the 2 tips that you can take advantage to know them more.

- *Most of the time we are not noticing that we already have been bitten by insects. Since a portion of the insects that we have in the world today like the Anopheles Malaria mosquitoes don't produce sounds and don't leave an imprint in the wake of its presence.*

- *If you were bitten by an insect which resulted in an infection, sometimes symptoms will not show up. In some cases, you may even have a mellow type of sickness and may feel that you simply have influenza or a cold, or even an undesirable skin rash.*

Hazard factors

In case you work outside or regularly participate in open air exercises, for example, outdoors or climbing, you are inclined to be at risk of insect bites. Since most of the time, the outside dress should be comfortable that is why we used to wear shorts which reveal a large segment of our skin, for example, legs and arms, that gives you a higher risk of getting bitten by insects.

When would it be advisable for me to see a medical professional?

See your doctor in the event that you have serious manifestations (for instance, in the event that you have a ton of swelling and pain) or if there is discharge, which demonstrates an infection.

Chapter 2 – Natural Mosquito Repellent Recipes

Mosquitoes are normally less dynamic toward the beginning of the day as they can't withstand the beams of the sun. Actually, they may even get got dried out and die when exposed to an excessive amount of daylight. However, it is a completely different story at night.

The minute the sun starts to set, mosquitoes start their chase for their next host, would you like to avoid them in the most ideal and regular way? Then the use of natural insect repellents will save you all the way from the irritation and illnesses that mosquito bites can bring.

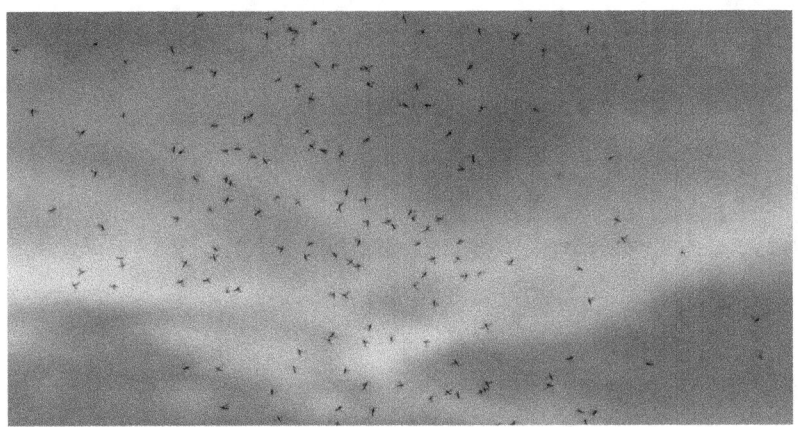

Lemon Eucalyptus Oil

Ingredients:

Lemon eucalyptus oil - 10 milliliters

Coconut or olive oil - 90 milliliters

Instructions:

- *Get a 100 milliliters jug and pour 10 milliliters of lemon eucalyptus oil to it.*

- *Put 90 milliliters of either coconut or olive oil to the lemon eucalyptus oil and blend them carefully.*

- *Apply this blend generously to the affected region.*

How Many Times Should You Apply This?

Reapply this blend intermittently, particularly when you are outside.

Why this is Effective?

Lemon eucalyptus oil contains mixes like citronellal and p-methane 3,8-diol (PMD). While citronellal is accepted to demonstrate a little repellency against mosquitoes, PMD is profoundly powerful against these insects that are considered as pests.

Peppermint Oil and Coconut Oil

Ingredients:

Peppermint oil - 12 drops

Coconut oil - 30 milliliters

Instructions:

- *Mix peppermint oil with coconut oil.*

- *Apply this blend generously to your hands and legs.*

How Many Times You Should Do This

Execute this 2-3 times before you go outside your house.

Why This is Effective?

Peppermint oil is a kind of essential oil that functions admirably in getting rid of mosquitoes. Consolidating it with coconut oil upgrades its mosquito repellent potential and essentially makes it your own one of a kind insect repellent. While peppermint contains mixes like limonene and menthol that keeps mosquitoes under control, coconut oil contains unsaturated fats and emulsifiers that hinder the vanishing of the anti-agents particles of peppermint oil.

Neem Oil and Coconut Oil

Ingredients

Neem oil - 9 drops

Coconut oil - 25 milliliters

Instructions:

- *Put the neem oil to coconut oil.*

- *Mix well and apply this generously to the uncovered areas of your body.*

How Many Times You Should Do This?

Apply this, at any amount, two times per day.

Why This Works?

Neem oil is gotten from the seeds and products of the neem tree. It is accepted to have normal mosquito repellent properties because of its attributes and solid smell. Truth be told, an investigation has demonstrated that 2% neem oil, when utilized in mix with coconut oil, gave huge protection guaranteed against various types of mosquitoes.

Citronella Oil And Alcohol Spray

Ingredients:

Liquor - 10 milliliters

Citronella oil - 10 drops

Water - 80 milliliters

Instructions:

- *Blend liquor and water in predetermined extents.*

- *Include citronella oil and blend well.*

- *Put this in a small container and splash on the uncovered areas of your body.*

How Many Times You Should Do This?

You should do this 2 to multiple times day by day before you head outside.

Why This Works?

Citronella oil is acquired from the leaves of the lemongrass plant. It contains numerous mixes like citronellal, geraniol, citronellol, citral, and limonene that display mosquito repellent properties.

Soda With Vinegar Mosquito Trap

Ingredients:

1 cup of vinegar

1/4 cup of soft drinks

Instructions:

- *Get an empty jug and cut it into half.*

- *Put the soft drink to the base part of the jug.*

- *Take the top piece of the jug and transform it with the goal that it would look like a channel.*

- *Place the modified portion of the container over the half of the base.*

- *Pour vinegar into this and spot it outside your room.*

How Many Times You Should Do This

Do this at whatever point there is an expansion in the number of mosquitoes in your general vicinity.

Why This Works?

When there is the presence of soft drinks that interacts with vinegar, the response between the two discharges carbon dioxide. Carbon dioxide pulls in mosquitoes and consequently can be utilized to trap and kill them.

Chapter 3 – Bed Bug Repellent Recipes

Homemade Bug Spray

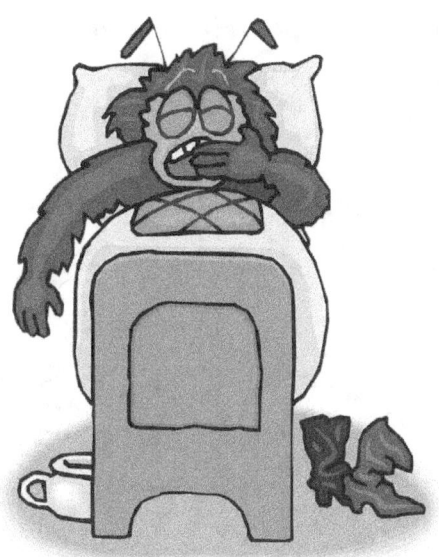

Ingredients:

Geranium essential oil – 29 drops

Citronella essential oil – 29 drops

Lemon eucalyptus essential oil – 19 drops

Lavender essential oil – 19 drops

Rosemary essential oil – 9 drops

Vodka or rubbing alcohol – 1 tablespoon

Natural witch hazel – half cup

Water or vinegar – half cup

Instructions

- *Put the essential oils in a <u>glass spray container.</u> Include vodka or other types of alcoholic drinks and shake tremendously for it to combine well.*

- *Add the witch hazel and shudder it to mix well.*

- *If preferred put half teaspoon of vegetable glycerin. This is not mandatory however helps the ingredients to stay intact.*

- *Include water and shake repeatedly. Shake every after use as the oils and water will naturally split eventually.*

How to Use

I place the container on my cabinet for easy access, and also in our first aid kit whenever I am going outdoors. I also bring with me my personally made cream for itching to protect me from bug bites.

<u>Herbal Bug Spray</u>

What do you need?

- ✓ *Water (must be distilled)*
- ✓ *Rubbing alcohol*
- ✓ *Peppermint*
- ✓ *Citronella*
- ✓ *Catnip*
- ✓ *Lavender*
- ✓ *Spearmint*
- ✓ *Lemongrass*

What to do?

- *Heat a cup of water and put 2-3 tbsp of herbs total in any mixture from the ingredients above. I utilize 1 tbsp each of spearmint, citronella, and lemongrass, and also put in some cloves preferably the dry ones.*
- *Combine carefully, coat and let the heat subside.*
- *Remove the water from the herbs and put it in a cup of witch hazel or rubbing alcohol.*
- *Pour in a spray container in a humid area. It is advisable to keep it in the fridge for maximal preservation.*
- *Use as necessary.*

Essential oils

Thyme, lemongrass, lavender, and tea tree oils can be utilized to diminish bed bugs for good. Basically blend five to ten drops of these with water, empty it into a spray container and splash on the surfaces that are necessary to be sprayed. It can both repulse and slaughter bed bugs as a result of its normal properties. It can likewise be utilized on the body as an anti-agents, yet the centralization of the essential oils ought to be almost no for that utilization.

Rubbing Alcohol

In the event that you tapped the connection above about the potential for causing a flame with hand-crafted insect repellent, at that point you will realize that rubbing alcohol was somewhat in charge of the blast. That doesn't need to stop you, be that as it may, from using this personally made solution.

The motivation behind why the general population in that news report had their home burst into flames is on the grounds that they were utilizing alcohol close to open fire, so simply recall that significant wellbeing tip on an instance that you choose to utilize this technique. Try not to utilize alcohol on close flame or notwithstanding consuming incense.

Chapter 4 – Lice Repellent Recipes

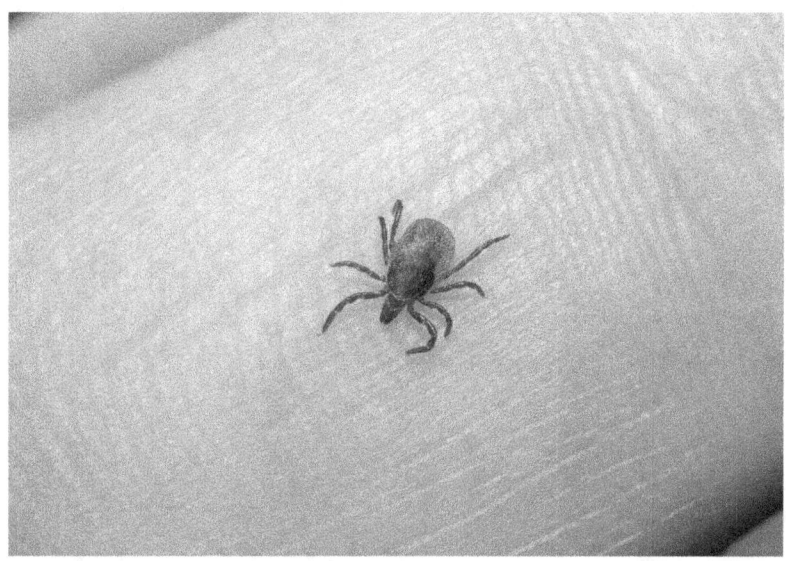

Recipe #1

Blend the accompanying essential oils in a 3 ounces spray container, filled most of the way with water. In case that you have a much larger container, modify the essential oil sum as needs be.

What do you need?

- ✓ *Tea tree oil - 9 drops*

- ✓ *Lavender oil - 4 drops*

- ✓ *Rosemary oil - 4 drops*

- ✓ *Peppermint oil - 4 drops*

Shake a long time before you use it and rest assured that those nasty lice will be off the hook!

Recipe #2

- ✓ *Water - 5 oz.*

- ✓ *Vodka - 5 oz.*

- ✓ *Essential oils - 79 drops*

- ✓ *Neem oil - 2 teaspoons*

- ✓ Blend the majority of the oils in an 8 ounces spray container.

- ✓ Shake the container and spray on hair every morning, and again when going to places where lice presentation is likely!

As a model, for my last shower, I add more oils, and after that increased the alcohol content to help diminish them. I combined the accompanying: 2 teaspoons of neem oil a couple of squirts of argan oil, 29 drops tea tree essential oil, 19 drops eucalyptus essential oil, 19 drops lavender, 5 drops cinnamon leaf oil, 4 drops geranium oil.

At that point filled the container with more vodka, alongside a dash of refined water, and shook it to consolidate everything really well. In the event that you are utilizing for youngsters under 10, you can supplant the eucalyptus oil with an alternative oil on the rundown, or a blend of oils.

Recipe #3

What do you need?

- ✓ *Water - 2 oz.*

- ✓ *Tea tree oil - 11 drops*

- ✓ *Spray container – this sort of plastic container is likely a decent alternative too.*

- ✓ *Lavender oil - 5 drops (either Hungarian or Bulgarian)*

Technique

- o Mix the above ingredients in the spray container and splash on hair.

- o No compelling reason to rinse it out.

- o To Prevent Lice: Spray on hair day by day toward the beginning of the day or potentially around evening time. Work through the whole head of hair.

- o To Remove Lice: Spray on the hair around evening time and search over hosed hair with absolute attention to detail toward the beginning of the day.

Quick Notes: Hungarian Lavender has a sweet aroma, and Bulgarian Lavender has an increasingly herbaceous fragrance. So pick depending on your preference.

Neem Oil Shampoo

Neem oil, similar to tea tree oil, is likewise viewed as a common insect spray. Numerous botanists use it to diminish bugs in their nurseries. It is successful yet it has a dreadful smell.

Add a couple of teaspoons to your ordinary cleanser (plain cleanser, not molding) or some unscented fluid Castile cleanser to make a neem oil cleanser.

Apple Cider Vinegar

Is there anything apple juice vinegar isn't useful for? On an instance that there is, I don't think I've discovered it. When you cleanse, wash your hair with apple juice vinegar. Or then again simply douse your hair with ACV, let it sit for a couple of minutes and after that brush out your hair with a nit brush.

Essential Oil Treatment

- ✓ *Sesame seed oil - 1/4 cup*
- ✓ *Neem oil - 1/8 cup*
- ✓ *Tea tree basic oil - 11 drops*
- ✓ *Eucalyptus oil - 6 drops*
- ✓ *Rosemary basic oil - 4 drops*
- ✓ *Lavender essential oil - 9 drops*

Soak hair with apple juice vinegar and apply the oil blend to your hair.

Spread it with a shower top and leave it in for 6 or 8 hours (think about it in the event that you don't have time amid the day).

Search over with a nit brush the following morning and cleanser as you ordinarily would. Utilize this treatment consistently for the multi-week basis to dispose of head lice.

Epsom Salt and Water

When you mix it with water may get dried out and diminish lice. To utilize, apply 2-3 tablespoons Epsom salt broke down in 1/4 container warm water (or more if necessary) to the scalp/hair. Enable the solution to sit until the hair is completely dry, at that point wash before beginning with Step 1.

Coconut Or Olive Oil and Essential Oils

As referenced above, in this investigation, a cream that included 10% tea tree and 1% lavender oil was 97.6% powerful in disposing of lice, while bug sprays like pyrethrins and piperonyl butoxide were just 25% successful.

Chapter 5 – Additional Insect Repellent Recipes

Vodka Surprise – Spray On

To start with, blend everything aside from the essential oils. When the base is in, include the oils and shake well for quick use!

What do you need?

- ✓ *Witch hazel - 3 tbsp.*
- ✓ *Almond oil, jojoba oil, or avocado oil. - 3 tbsp.*
- ✓ *Vodka - half tsp.*
- ✓ *Lemon eucalyptus essential oil - 54 drops*
- ✓ *Lavender oil essential oil - 16 drops*
- ✓ *Cedarwood essential oil - 14 drops*
- ✓ *Rosemary essential oil - 14 drops*
- ✓ *Spray container - 9 ounces*

Skin Smoothing – Spray On

Essentially combine the majority of the ingredients, shake, and shower! The skin relieving benefits originate from both witch hazel and apple juice vinegar. Numerous sorts of toner and other great items to help prevent skin break out, perspiring, razor consumes, and the sky is the limit from there!

What do you need?

- ✓ *Apple juice vinegar - half cup*
- ✓ *Witch hazel - half cup*
- ✓ *Eucalyptus - 39 drops*
- ✓ *Spray container - 9 ounces*

Non-Edible Alcohol – Spray On

Include the majority of the essential oils into a spray container, and afterward include liquor and shake. After these ingredients consolidate, put in the witch hazel and give it another great shake!

What do you need?

1. *Rubbing alcohol - 1 tablespoon*
2. *Witch hazel - half cup*
3. *Glycerin - 1 teaspoon*
4. *Water or vinegar - half cup*
5. *Geranium essential oil - 29 drops*
6. *Citronella essential oil - 29 drops*
7. *Lavender essential oil - 19 drops*
8. *Lemon eucalyptus essential oil – 21 drops*
9. *Rosemary essential oil - 9 drops*
10. *Spray bottle - 9 ounces*

Simple Essentials Homemade Insect Repellent – Rub On

What do you need?

1. *Transporter oil of your preference (avocado oil, grapeseed oil, coconut oil) - 2 tablespoon*

2. *The essential oil of your choice - 20 drops*

3. *Spray container*

Add the transporter oil to your container, and afterward blend in the essential oils. Shake before you rub this oil blend onto your skin!

Water-based Combination Insect Repellent – Spray-on

What do you need?

1. *Lemon juice - 3-4 tablespoons*

2. *Lavender essential oil - 14 drops*

3. *Vanilla concentrate - 3-4 tablespoon*

4. *Distilled water*

Consolidate all the ingredients in your preferred spray container, and shake.In the event that you would prefer not to buy refined water, just bubble water for a similar impact.

The Easiest Essential Oil Recipe – Rub On or Spray On

What do you need?

- ✓ *Lemon eucalyptus essential oil*

- ✓ *Choose either one of the following: Witch hazel, sunflower oil, neem oil, and almond oil.*

Blend 1 part of the essential oil with 11 drops of the witch hazel or oil. To blend it up, have a go at utilizing more than one kind of oil!

Smell Like a Mosquito Repelling Candle – Rub On

What do you need?

- *Citronella essential oil - 11 drops*

- *Eucalyptus essential oil - 11 drops*

- *Cedar fundamental oil - 5 drops*

- *Your preferred oil (jojoba, neem, and fennel) - 4 tablespoons*

Bugs Hate Mouthwash – Spray On

What do you need?

1. *A mouthwash of your choice*

2. *1 spray container*

Just shower mouthwash on yourself as a simple personally-made insect repellent. Always remember despite that it is a mouthwash you should not drink it because we already transformed it into an insect repellent, just be cautious with that to prevent any unwanted incidents that might happen.

Zest Cabinet Raid – Spray On

What do you need?

1. *Water - 1 cup*

2. *Witch hazel or rubbing alcohol - 1 cup*

3. *Dried herbs any of the following: peppermint, lavender, catnip, or spearmint - 4 tablespoons*

4. *Dried cloves - 2 pieces*

5. *Spray container*

Consolidate the water, herbs, and cloves then heat to the point of boiling. When it is already heated, fill the container, blend, spread, and let the solution cool totally. At the point when the mix is cool, strain the herbs and throw them away. Keep the water and include the rest of the ingredients, witch hazel or rubbing alcohol. Store this handcrafted creepy crawly repellent in a cool spot like the icebox.

Castile Soap Soup – Spray On

What do you need?

1. *Fluid Castile cleanser - 9 teaspoon*

2. *Neem oil - 1 teaspoon*

3. *Refined water - 4 containers*

4. *Spray bottle - 1 piece*

Consolidate all the ingredients, shake, and apply!

The Marinator – Spray On

The marinator is known for the smelliest handcrafted bug repellent formula that is around for a long time. In any case, as it dries the smell disperses to people. To ticks and mosquitoes, this stuff keeps directly on smelling and annoying for them resulting in a total diminishing of them!

What do you need?

1. *Dried sage - 2 tablespoons*

2. *Thyme - 2 tablespoons*

1. *Mint - 2 tablespoons*

2. *Rosemary - 2 tablespoons*

3. *Lavender - 2 tablespoons*

4. *Apple juice vinegar - 32 ounces*

5. *Spray bottles*

Blend all the ingredients in the glass container. Seal well, and put it in a place you won't neglect to shake day by day. Shake well each day for 2-3 weeks.

After this tincture has had sufficient energy to marinate, strain the herbs and keep everything in the fridge. Since this stuff is so incredible, blend a balance of the blend and water in the splash bottles.

Peppermint and Vanilla Tincture – Spray On

What do you need?

1. *Vodka - 1 container*

2. *Vanilla concentrate - 1 tablespoon*

3. *Cloves - 1 tablespoon*

4. *Peppermint extricate - 1 tablespoon*

5. *Spray bottle*

Consolidate everything into the container, shake, and let it sit for a while. This custom made bug repellent works better the more it is permitted to sit as long as a month. In case you go this course, try to shake day by day. Note: you may need to strain out the cloves in the wake of soaking.

The Italian Job – Spray On

What do you need?

1. *Refined water - half container*

2. *Vodka - half container*

3. *Cleaved crisp basil - 1 container*

4. *spray bottle - 1 piece*

Convey water to a moving bubble, and include the basil. Heat this blend to the point of boiling, spread, and let sit for at least 6 hours. At the point when time is up, strain out the herbs and empty the fragrant water into the shower bottle. Include vodka, shake, and your natively constructed bug repellent is prepared to go!

Vanilla Extract – Spray On or Rub On

The vanilla concentrate can be added to any of the plans of the trivial oil for included security. Moreover, it can really be utilized without anyone else to repulse mosquitoes. Rub it on the skin, or blend it with a balance of witch hazel and water for a brisk, tyke well disposed, and shower capable form. It is also known that vanilla is great for the skin because it has properties that nourish and brings suppleness to our skin.

So you are hitting to birds in one stone, you are protecting yourself from the harmful effects of insect bites and at the same time enhance your appearance. Do not hesitate now and try this recipe out and you will surely know what I am talking about. This is probably the best for you if you are looking to have a good lotion and insect repellent in an all-in-one action.

Conclusion

Wow, that was a great learning experience for all of us. We had able to learn the different insect repellents to keep us safe at all times. Aside from that upon bringing those recipes to life you will gain a lot of benefits from it such as you will not get any side-effects because the ingredients are all natural.

The good thing with the recipes that we discussed is that you will save a lot of money as well from buying ready-made insect repellents in the market minus the artificial ingredients that can impose a significant risk in our health in the form of cancers, allergies, and many more than you can ever imagine.

One suggestion that I can give you is after you have created the certain insect repellent recipe from this book, try a small portion first on your skin before applying it generously. This will help you see if the recipe is compatible with your skin.I am not saying that because the recipes are all-natural you will not take any precautionary measures at all, it is always better to be safe at all times.

Although some of the recipes that I have included here obviously does not smell well because its primary purpose is to repel those unwanted insects away from you. However, you can also blend the recipes with the essential oils of your choice to make them smell more pleasing.

As far as I can remember I have experimented some and found significant success on it. The good thing is the recipes smelled better and at the same time did not lose their effectiveness in chasing away insects.

Since then those recipes became a part of my daily routine right now I am really happy that I have the confidence that I and my family are safe from the harmful effects of insect bites. As you have read in this book a while ago the different recipes that you can use to repel different kinds of insects and as a beginner, you will notice that the recipes that I have included are composed of the user-friendly ones and the more complex recipes.

My advice starts first with the simple recipes from there you will have the chance to get a glimpse of how to blend properly. So once you mastered blending you can level up by creating the much more complex recipes and practice it very often so that the next time that you will be doing it you will become more comfortable.

That's it! I hope you enjoyed this book and I suggest that you refer this book to your friends after you read it because it is always a good decision to become protected from insect bites. As the world evolves, a new strain of diseases that is transferrable through a bite of an insect is truly frightening. The pieces of knowledge that you have found here are truly priceless. Why? Because you cannot put a price on the health of you and your family.

Debra Hill

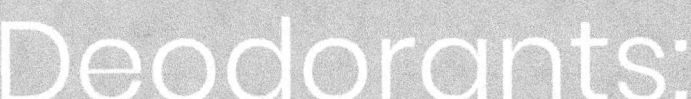

Deodorants:

Easy Recipes For Fresh and Effective Deodorants

Deodorants:
Easy Recipes For Fresh and Effective Deodorants

Introduction

When I was still a child I am not experiencing any kinds of bad odor especially on my armpit, it was only when I reached my adolescent stage when I experienced a significant change especially on my metabolism. I began to sweat more which is really a great deal on why I accumulated a bad odor especially on my armpit since then. I was frustrated and helpless because I have no idea on what to do in battling my bad odor problem. It was really a nightmare for me because I was bullied and I cannot do anything because what they are saying are all true.

I asked my mom on what do I need to do to combat the problem. She told me that I have to cleanse carefully my body especially the armpit when I am taking a bath and apply a deodorant afterward. I did the routines that my mom advice throughout the years until I became an adult however I am noticing that it has a lot of side-effects not only my skin but also on my overall wellness.

This is the primary reasons why I discovered that the artificial deodorant that I am using is composed of chemicals that are harmful to the health. This is where I had an urge to learn how to make natural deodorant recipes for personal use.

It truly changed my life for the better because it made myself healthier and most importantly free from bad odor. As time passed by, I realized that it wasn't enough for me to keep the knowledge by myself so I decided to share it to you on this book so that you will also have the ability to enjoy the privilege that I have.

Chapter 1 – Why Deodorants Are Important?

Imagine a situation where you enter a public vehicle, let's say a bus or train, or let's say a public place, and then there you are, you suddenly hold your breath or covered your nose for long because of that unwanted smell roaming around the place? Of course, you know that it came from someone's sweaty underarms and then you might say that "do they even use deodorant?" We all know that it is embarrassing especially if we are on that person's place.

But did you know that the sweat our body produces is odorless or close to it? Then you might ask: "Then where did that bad smell came from?" So let's start with it, our skin pores in the body produce sweat because of the waste that passes through it. The hotter the climate is the more sweat our body produces especially on the warm parts of our bodies, like for example, the underarms.

The bad smell that we all hate doesn't come from the sweat, but from bacteria that is on the sweat. There are a lot of people that use deodorant, and some use them almost every day and continues it for a long period of time where stopping the use if it will never be an option. There are also other people who don't really need these deodorants or simply does not use them at all, and believe me it is all fine. But for those who use deodorants, they don't really know that the effectiveness of it is just low.

We all know that the deodorant's purpose is to get rid of the body odor in us. And yes it is the main reason and the only reason we have that's why we use deodorants. There is something like deodorant that is called "Antiperspirants", but they function differently. Antiperspirants keep us from producing body odor thus making us smell fresh, and they stop our sweat glands to produce too much sweat.

But take note that antiperspirants don't really work, I mean, like the deodorant, its effectiveness is low because there will be a time that our body will reject and become immune from the effects of the antiperspirant.

Like you, I am also curious about how exactly deodorants get rid of the bad smell our body have. In all honesty, both things, the deodorant, and antiperspirants are quite complicated. But here today, I'll be listing down some of the effects of deodorants on our body.

3. Deodorants eliminate those odor-causing bacteria

Like what I've just said earlier, sweat is almost completely odorless, because there are some studies that proved sweat is nearly odorless. Body odor comes out when the body's bacteria breaks down one of two types of sweat. That only means, the bad smell that we usually produce from excessive sweating doesn't come out right after we sweat for a small amount, and if the sweat doesn't stay too long from your skin. So all in all, the main idea of deodorant is that they can kill the bacteria that causes bad odor, and that is all.

4. Deodorants do not stop you from sweating

Well, the daily use of deodorants and antiperspirants led some of us to believe that they both work the same way but in reality, they don't. Just like said recently, deodorants keep us from smelling bad, they get rid of the bacteria in the sweat, but they don't stop the sweat glands from producing sweat.

Now, on the other hand, the antiperspirants help to stop the production of excess sweat on the sweat glands in order to get rid of excessive and unwanted sweat, especially on the underarms.

So to sum it all up, we put our money on the antiperspirants as they can help you get rid of this annoying extra sweat the same time maintain you smelling fresh, but do keep in mind that they only decrease the sweat glands production of sweat by only 20%.

5. *Use of deodorant can change the bacteria in the body*

There is a study that stated, the use of deodorants and antiperspirants can change the skin microbiome, meaning that they can somehow affect the bacteria in our body. In this study conducted, there were 17 persons where they are examined for about eight days. The researchers swabbed each of the person's underarms.

The first day of the study, the participants of the study does their standard underarm hygiene routine. Starting the second day up to the sixth, they all stopped using antiperspirants and deodorants. And for the last two days, the seventh and eighth, all of them applied antiperspirants.

As for the final result, it has shown that everyone who participated in the study has an increase of bacteria on their underarms the time they stopped using the antiperspirants and deodorants.

6. *Use of deodorant can lead to breast cancer*

Some might say that women who use deodorants and antiperspirants every day can increase the chances of them having breast cancer in the future. This may bother some of you, but here is an explanation of why it is not true. There is a theory that stated, the aluminum in the antiperspirants and the parabens in the deodorants can produce some hormonal effects, estrogen-like.

These things can contribute in the growth of breast cancer cells and there are a few numbers of scientific studies that stated there is somehow a connection, but the FDA and the National Cancer Institute does not support this claims.

Now knowing this, we think that you should not be afraid of using deodorants and antiperspirants, why? It is because it is not proven that it can lead to breast cancer, and there are no cases which stated they developed breast cancer because they use deodorants and antiperspirants daily. There are still studies being conducted about these claims, and as long as it is not yet proven, the use of these products are completely safe.

Why Deodorants are very important for Women in Modern Life?

The use of antiperspirants and deodorants are very high especially on hotter places on earth, for one good reason, people there sweat a lot. And we have our own lives, we have our own jobs, and things we do, physically to be exact, and because of this, we also sweat a lot, like a lot. So how to deal with it?

Grab your deodorant or antiperspirant and your good to go. Well, believe it or not, but these products, the antiperspirants, and deodorants have been running all along the way back to the time of the Ancient Egyptians, well actually it started from them.

They experiment with different natural materials to use as scented products for the underarms, one example is cinnamon. But here in our modern world, most antiperspirants and deodorants contain chemicals in order for a better and likable result.

A lot of us are annoyed when we sweat especially when you are working on an office or a place that is air-conditioned because when the bad odor starts to kick in, it will just spread out in the whole place and the smell will just stay there and somehow will leave a dark spot in your shirt near the underarms. It is just embarrassing, right? But you should know that sweating is actually good for the body.

Sweating is a normal thing that happens in the body, it is a natural way of cooling our bodies when it is hot. So come to think about what happens when you stop it. That is what happens every single time you use an antiperspirant. So it is still important to put the balance on things and try not to use them daily.

Well, having some knowledge about deodorants and antiperspirants can be good, but what if you process more info about it? Like for example, did you know that we spend almost $18 billion dollars a year for these products, just for the sake of removing bad odors or making your sweat glands stop producing sweat? Come think of that $18 billion dollars. And here, I'll be listing down some of the things that you might not know about antiperspirants and deodorants.

6. *Deodorant eliminates bacteria*

Well, we all know that the one that causes those bad odors are the bacteria on the sweat, right? So here is the deodorant coming up to save the day. They will keep you smelling good as they eliminate those bacteria that lies in your sweat.

7. *The anti-body odor is an old-time trend*

Yes, you heard that right. Like said from the previous one up there, the Ancient Egyptians made the first anti-body odor products which are later known as deodorants.

And did you know that the first ever trademarked deodorant is called Mum and was created in 1888, man that is a long time ago. And after 15 years, the first ever antiperspirant came out and it is called Everdry.

8. *Antiperspirants do not really stop the production of sweat.*

This aluminum found in antiperspirants does a good job of stopping the eccrine sweat glands. But it is just 20 percent effective.

9. *Your body can become immune to the antiperspirant you use daily*

Believe it or not but our bodies can adapt to the effects an antiperspirant can do to our sweat glands, and no one knows how can this happen. Some said that the body can find its own way of resisting the effects and starts to produce more sweat on other glands. A doctor said that it is better to have a variety of brands for deodorants and antiperspirants in order to prevent the body to adapt from its effects.

10. Whether you're a man or woman, deodorant is effective

Do you know that women have more sweat glands than men? Yes, it's true but the cool thing here is men's sweat glands produces more sweat then women do. Although there are separate products or brands of antiperspirants and deodorants that are specified for men and women, in reality, they are all the same, and all of these "separated" things is just a marketing strategy. And it is funny to think that all of us still falls for this kind of marketing. The only thing that differs is the style and scent of the deodorant.

11. *Some people do not need deodorants*

Well, some may advertise really well that people are still convinced to buy and use deodorants every day. And do you know that most people don't smell bad at all? Yes, it is all true. And some people are simply lucky because they naturally don't smell bad at all because of their genes.

12. *No one really knows where those yellow stains came from*

Not even the ones who make deodorants and antiperspirants and not even the scientists know why are there yellow stains left in the underarms when they use deodorants and antiperspirants.

But the main thing here is that some theorize that it came from the aluminum compounds which can be seen on antiperspirants as they have certain chemical reactions with the sweat, shirt or the skin. And according to some research, the best way to get rid of these yellow stains is just to simply avoid buying and using aluminum-based antiperspirants.

13. *You can produce your own deodorant and antiperspirant*

Isn't that amazing that you can improvise or somehow create your own deodorant and antiperspirant right at your own home! Well, there are certain things or ingredients needed in order to make one.

The bright side of making your own deodorant or antiperspirant is that it is very easy to do, and for the brighter side of it, it can cost you less or nothing at all because they are purely natural, all you need is some certain oil and extracts together with its antibacterial compounds which can add up in removing those unwanted bad smell from your underarm.

Chapter 2 – Artificial Versus Natural Deodorants

Starting with this topic, I'll give you the things you must know in order to understand what is in between these two types of deodorants and how they completely differ from each other. So first things first, what is an artificial deodorant? It is obvious, right?

An artificial deodorant is made up of chemicals and partly natural ingredient. On the other hand, is the All-Natural Deodorant, well we also know that this is very obvious, it all tells it by its name. These deodorants are all made from natural and organic materials or ingredients in order to make those scented anti-bacterial bad odor removing deodorants.Now that I gave you a head start in today's topic, I will be listing down the things you must know why you should switch from artificial deodorant into natural ones. But first why?

In reality, we can use those artificially made deodorants in general but you might want to know that these deodorants don't work at all for some people, because sometimes their body resists these product's effectiveness.

You might be one of these people and in order for you to have a working deodorant product, you might want to try being all-natural in this situation, what I mean is start researching about certain ingredients you can use in making your own natural deodorant that will perfectly work on your body and can adapt on your sweat glands. So now I will be listing down the reasons why you should use natural deodorants than artificial ones.

11. Artificial deodorants do contain ingredients that can be harmful to your health

So here we are again talking about the risks of using deodorants and antiperspirants. There is a study that proved, using aluminum-based antiperspirants can increase the chance of having an Alzheimer's disease by 60 percent.

And yet the theory of increasing the chance of having breast cancer by using aluminum-based antiperspirants are here again although this claim about cancer is not yet proven, why not just become safe and try to change your old aluminum-based antiperspirant into a not aluminum based one right?

12. Natural deodorants have ingredients that are good for your body

There are natural deodorants that contain charcoal on it, and for you to know, it is not only the natural deodorants that use charcoal but also other cosmetic products. So what does this charcoal do exactly?

It helps absorbs moisture more than you can think of and wait for it, the best part is when charcoal is ingested, it can help you with gastrointestinal problems, can you believe that? Can your recent artificial deodorant do that? There are some plant-based deodorants that can help your underarms to stay fresh and smooth. These ingredients are olive oil, clay-rich in mineral, and Shea butter.

They help make your underarms to become smooth and irritation free. When your underarms do not irritate from the artificial products you use, underarm shaves can last longer. And there are some other ingredients that can help smoothen out razor burns and shrink pores.

The good thing about these natural deodorants is that they don't block the pores in our skin unlike what the antiperspirants do. What these natural deodorant do is they let the good bacteria do their own thing on your skin which is to help lessen the odor.

Because like said previously, it is not the sweat that causes the bad odor, the odor only comes out when the bacteria mixes with your sweat. That's why using natural deodorants can help you get rid of this bacteria, making you smell good.

13. *Does detoxification happen whenever you switch from artificial to natural deodorant?*

There is one statement that said they don't believe in a detoxification period once you switched from artificial to natural deodorant. They stated that once you use the natural one, it will immediately work on the spot.

But for those first timers in using natural deodorants, they must understand that the effectiveness of it still depends on a person's way of living, the food he or she eats and his or her daily physical activities and many more. You must also take note that an aluminum-free deodorant doesn't stop sweat at all.

Those only with ingredients that are safe for you will just help stop the bad odor but they won't keep you dry for the whole day, I mean, they won't keep you dry at all. Just don't stop the sweating, it is not harmful and like said, the sweat is not the one that causes the bad odor, but the bacteria mixed on it. In reality, sweating is a sign that your body is healthy. Don't you want that?

Based on my study, some said that the best way to make the most out of your deodorant is to balance how much you use it. Some people claimed that one or two swipes of deodorants helped them stayed odorless the whole day. And please keep in mind that unlike the artificial deodorants, natural ones only need small amounts to be applied to your underarm in order to work.

Things You Must Know about the Natural and Artificial Deodorants

Of course, you are here for a reason, and that is to know how does these two differ? What are their advantages on each other, disadvantages? And yeah, you are finding the one that will best suit your situation, or in other words, you are finding what product will work best for your body.

It is common for us that we always find precautionary measures in order to be safe from the products that we are going to use.

Well, in this part of the article, I'll be answering down the most common questions asked by people about natural deodorants and artificial deodorants. Stay tuned, you might find the answer you've been looking for here.

4. *Are deodorants and antiperspirants the same?*

For a simpler explanation, the antiperspirants work is to stop the sweat glands from producing sweat, well in reality, not stop at all but reduces its production, while the deodorant, on the other hand, stops that annoying bad odor that lingers around whenever your underarms sweat. Although antiperspirants are also deodorants, not all deodorants are antiperspirants. Think of it as an additional feature for deodorant.

5. *So which one stands out?*

So starting off, antiperspirants stop our sweat glands from sweating right? I believe that you know sweating is a part of the body's process, and it is a sign of healthiness. Sweating is the body's natural way of ventilation. A doctor said that if you don't sweat (naturally), it is a sign that your body can't or doesn't release the toxins inside that can be harmful to us or it is that you are having a bad metabolism.

The aluminum compound in the antiperspirant is an actual aluminum, and it is the most bothering ingredient this product has. So how does this work basically? These small aluminum compounds find their way to block those cells and pores on the skin thus making it look like your sweat glands stopped from producing sweat.

The use of aluminum products like utensils and other stuff has become controversial over the years, and I think that it goes the same with the deodorant. We must stop using aluminum-based antiperspirants. Because long-term use of this aluminum based product can cause serious damage to our tissues.

There is a study that shows aluminum are neurotoxins and can contribute massively to the production of breast cancer cells (the reason why aluminum-based antiperspirants are linked to breast cancer). Not just that, but it can also make the chances of having an Alzheimer's disease high and can cause toxicity in the liver.

Someone said that the use of antiperspirants depends on the person's need. Although the use of antiperspirants is commonly linked with breast cancer, one person stated that the aluminum compounds in the antiperspirants are too small for our body to absorb it completely and cause serious damage inside.

Because studies are still being conducted about the link of antiperspirants on breast cancer, if they are really connected, or if that antiperspirants really cause estrogen to change causing breast cancer cells to increase in amount.

But in order for you to find out what's best for your skin, I suggest that you look at the ingredients of the product you are going to buy.Look if there are common components that can cause skin irritation, these ingredients, for example, are the following propylene glycol, formaldehyde, geraniol, linalool, carboxaldehyde, benzyl salicylate.

And if you are deciding on what type of deodorant to buy, if it's a roll-on, stick, cream or spray. I suggest using the first three and try to avoid sprays, why? Deodorants are meant for skin, not the lungs. It is better to be safe.

6. *Any tips on how can I switch from one product to another?*

Well, made up your mind already in changing up your old deodorant? But do keep in mind that before starting a new one you must know that it will change your body care routine. Some of the natural deodorant users suggest that you detoxify your underarms first right after you get rid of your old deodorant. And I also believe that this is essential, it is because the detoxification will remove the excess chemicals your old deodorant had left on your underarms.

Think of this as a new fresh start, then right after you've detoxified your underarms, you can now start with your new deodorant brand. There is a simple mask you can make right at your house for this underarm detoxification, all you need is to mix up these ingredients with water: bentonite clay, apple cider, and vinegar.Well if you are not a fan of that detoxification thing, don't worry.

There is a statement that said our body has a natural way of detoxification, and yes I think you already know what that is already. Yes, of course, sweating. Being part of the natural processes of the body, there is no need to worry from chemicals harming you.

When you already started to use your all new natural deodorant and noticed that it is not working at all, you might want to try to exfoliate your underarms once a week. To do these, all you need is a washcloth then mix it up with oat flour and then unscented oil like coconut oil, then you're good to go.

Now that some of your questions are answered, now I will be listing down the reasons why you should avoid artificial deodorants and antiperspirants and start using natural deodorants now. Is it already obvious that all thing that is natural can benefit us a lot than those with chemical. But why do we keep on patronizing this artificial product? Is it because it is easy to buy?

Saves us time in preparing our own because these artificial ones are pre-made already? Yes, these reasons are also beneficial, but come think of this, is it beneficial for your own health? For me, I don't think so. That is why the best way to stay healthy, fresh and odor free, is to get rid of these artificial deodorants and antiperspirants and start using pure natural deodorants and antiperspirants.

Don't mind the time for preparation and the ingredients, because in the end it will be all worth it. So here are the reasons why you should give up your present artificial deodorant and antiperspirant.

5. *Artificial deodorants and antiperspirants contain harmful ingredients*

Yes that is right. It is mentioned a lot in this article, especially the antiperspirant having aluminum on its ingredients. So it is better to stay away from these chemical based products in order to reduce or the best, completely avoid complications in your body.

6. *Natural deodorants don't contain any aluminum*

Although artificial antiperspirants stop the sweat glands from sweating because of the aluminum ions that blocks it. Natural deodorants, on the other hand, work in a very different and safer way. There are compounds in the natural deodorants that help absorb wetness in the underarms effectively, these are plant-based powders and sodium bicarbonate or also known as baking soda.

7. *The scent of natural deodorants are also natural and chemical free*

What does this one mean? Artificial deodorants' scents contain a lot of chemicals in order to create that particular scent.

So imagine now the chemicals that flow right into your body. With the natural deodorants, it is all different, as it provides scent coming from essential oils which are all purely natural.

Chapter 3 – Amazing All-Natural Deodorant Recipes

We are close at the end of this article, and before we part ways, I would like to say thank you for staying until this part, so let us not waste some time, and let's get through this. Now, I will be listing down recipes that can help you make natural deodorants in your own house. I bet that you've read all the things that natural deodorant do? It is all beneficial rather than those artificial ones, right?

And I think that we must be concerned about the products we are using that is why I suggest that you do the natural ones as they don't contain harmful chemicals that artificial deodorants have. There is this ingredient in artificial deodorants called parabens, these include methyl, ethyl, propyl, benzyl, and butyl.

These ingredients are commonly found on the artificial deodorants you are using, and man, that is a lot of chemicals. And there are claims that these chemicals are linked also with breast cancer and other various diseases.

Here are some of the harmful chemicals or ingredients on artificial deodorants that you should avoid:

5. *Parabens (methyl, ethyl, propyl, benzyl, and butyl) - these chemicals are linked with breast cancer and other diseases.*
6. *Aluminum Compounds- often found in antiperspirants, these metallic materials are also linked with breast cancer.*
7. *Silica- These ingredients or chemicals are harmful to the body as they can contribute to cancer and allergies.*
8. *Triclosan- This ingredient is linked with cancer and skin irritations.*
9. *Talc- a chemical that is also linked with cancer.*

10. *Propylene Glycol- these chemicals are linked with liver and kidney problems and also allergic reactions.*
11. *Steareth-n- it is also linked with cancer.*

For the natural deodorant ingredients, here they are:

Homemade Deodorant for a Sensitive Skin

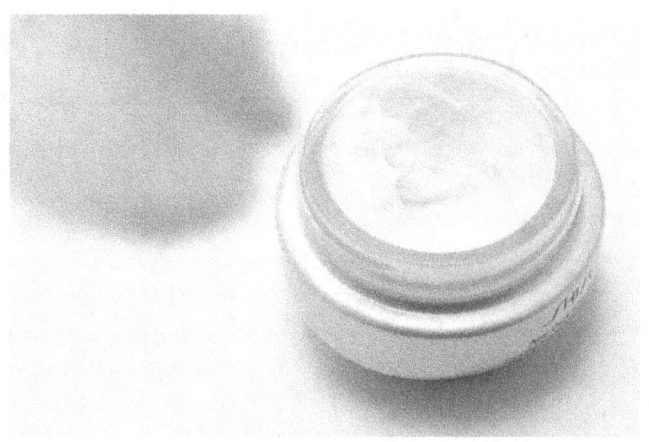

Ingredients:

3/4 cup arrowroot powder/non-GMO cornstarch
1/4 cup baking soda
4-6 tbsp. melted coconut oil

Procedure:

6. In a bowl, mix up the baking soda cornstarch or arrowroot powder
7. Then add up four tablespoons of melted coconut oil then mix. Keep on adding coconut oil until desired consistency is achieved.
8. Put the mixture into a jar with a tight cover.

Shea Butter Deodorant

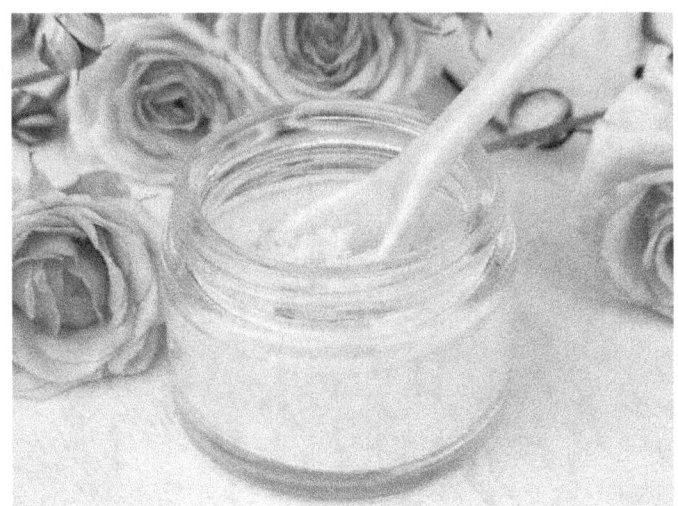

Ingredients:

3 tbsp. coconut oil

3 tbsp. baking soda

2 tbsp. shea butter

2 tbsp. arrowroot (optional) or organic cornstarch

Essential oils (optional)

Procedure:

3. Start by melting the Shea butter and coconut oil in a boiler over medium heat or you can just combine the coconut oil and the Shea butter in a glass jar with a cover then place it over in a pan with water until it melts.

4. Remove from heat then add up the arrowroot or if you don't have arrowroot, add more baking soda.

5. Then add up the essential oils then put all the mixture in a glass container. Don't need to the refrigerator. But it is up to you if you want to put it in the fridge, just to make it hard quickly.

Essential Oil Deodorant

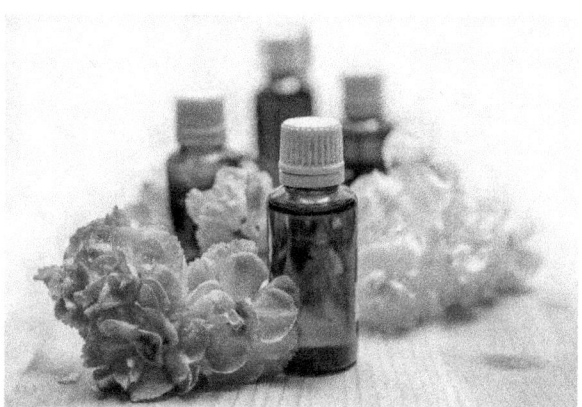

Ingredients:

2 1/2 tbsp. unrefined coconut oil

2 1/2 tbsp. unrefined shea butter

1/4 cup arrowroot starch/flour

2 tbsp. baking soda

6 drops lavender essential oil

6 drops grapefruit essential oil

2 drops tea tree essential oil (optional)

Procedure:

6. In a bowl or jar, put the coconut oil and Shea butter then place the bowl or jar in a medium pan.
7. Add water to the pan, just the right amount to surround the jar or bowl then boil it.
8. As it boils, continue to stir the coconut oil and Shea butter until it melts down.
9. Then right after, place it in separate jars (it is up to you what size) then put it in the fridge so that it will become hard quickly.
10. Make sure to keep the cover on when not in use.

Herbal Deodorant Spray

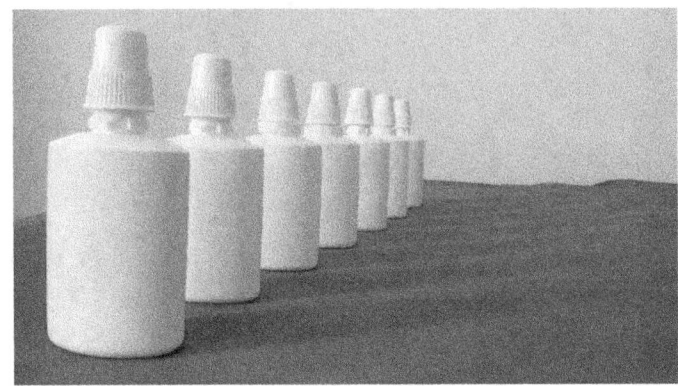

Ingredients:

1¼ cup 80 proof vodka

¼ cup sage leaves

¼ cup thyme leaves

¼ cup lavender buds

Peel of 1 lime or lemon

Essential oils:

Sage (6 drops)

Lavender (4 drops)

Tea tree (3 drops)

Patchouli (3 drops), and either lemongrass or lime(3 drops) per quarter-cup spray bottle

½ tsp. colloidal silver per quarter cup spray bottle, optional

Procedure:

5. In a pint-size jar, measure the herbs and citrus peels.
6. Pour vodka then cover it.
7. Keep the jar in a place where you can always find it, shake it once a day for about a month.

8. When the mixture is ready, funnel the liquid into a spray bottle.
9. Then add up the essential oil for fragrance.
10. Place the drained herbs somewhere you can find it until you are ready to use it again for another mixture.
11. Shake the spray bottle to mix up all the ingredients inside and not letting it only sit right on the top of the bottle.
12. Then you are good to go.

We've come the end of this article and I hope that you've learned a lot about deodorants and antiperspirants. This should give you the knowledge on what to use and how to use them.

To summarize them all, there are certain chemicals found in the ingredients of artificial deodorants and antiperspirants that can be extremely harmful to your health. So it is better to use the artificial ones as they give you the same results in a more safe way and much better.

Conclusion

There you have it, I hope that you have learned a lot from the wonderful deodorant recipes that are included in this book. Do not delay the action now and stop using artificial deodorants and starting switching to the natural ones that are included in the recipes that I mentioned on the previous chapters.

We therefore conclude that those recipes will bring us hundred folds of benefits that is why it is really necessary to put it on your daily routines. Be like me, because based on experience those recipes really improved myself not only my body odor, health, but also my confidence.

So if you want to improve your life for the better then take an action now. I wish you all the best in life!

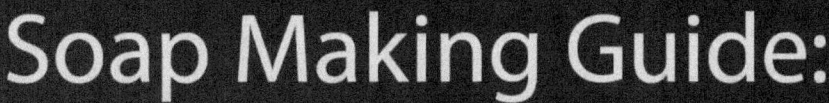

Soap Making Guide:

Beginner's Guide
To Making All-Natural, Mild Soap

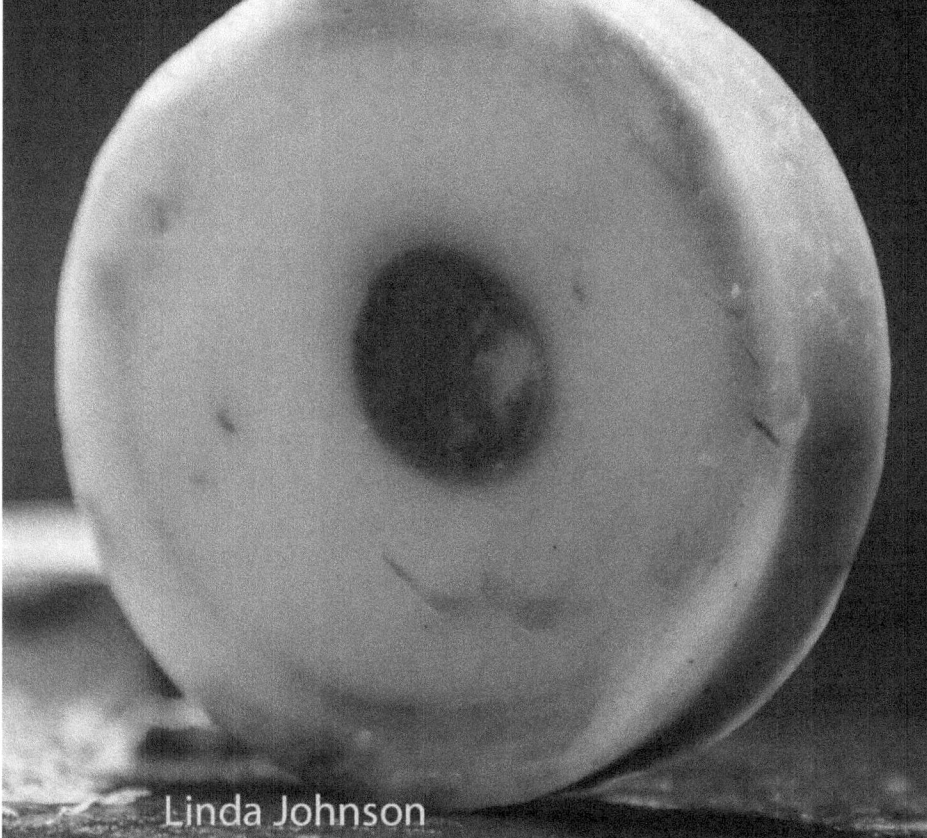

Linda Johnson

Soap Making Guide:

Beginner's Guide To Making All-Natural, Mild Soap

Introduction:

To give you a background about myself the journey of making soap is not that easy because I do not have the proper training in creating soaps beforehand that's why I urged myself to study and practice the craft tremendously until I mastered it. As time passes by, because of training and continued study on the craft I mastered it and in this book I will impart my knowledge to you regarding homemade soap making.

I realized that the knowledge must be shared because I have experienced a lot of benefits from it. Here are the following benefits that I got when I started using the soaps that I created:

- It made my skin smoother because the ingredients are all-natural which will not impose any risks on human's skin.

- My overall health significantly improved and I became more energized by using those soaps.

- Whenever I have a dilemma regarding my skin I just produce a particular soap that will help me solve the problem.

- I save a significant amount of money from buying soaps that I need on various purposes.

Chapter 1 – Different Kinds of Soaps

This is the thing we always use, what I mean is, this thing became part of our daily lives that some of us can't live without it. Can you believe that???! But yes it is true, soaps came from way back the 2800 BC, heck that was a long time ago! Soaps usually consist of natural oils mixed with sodium hydroxide and alkali, these ingredients are the reason why the soaps can clean our bodies effectively, leaving our skin a lot smoother.

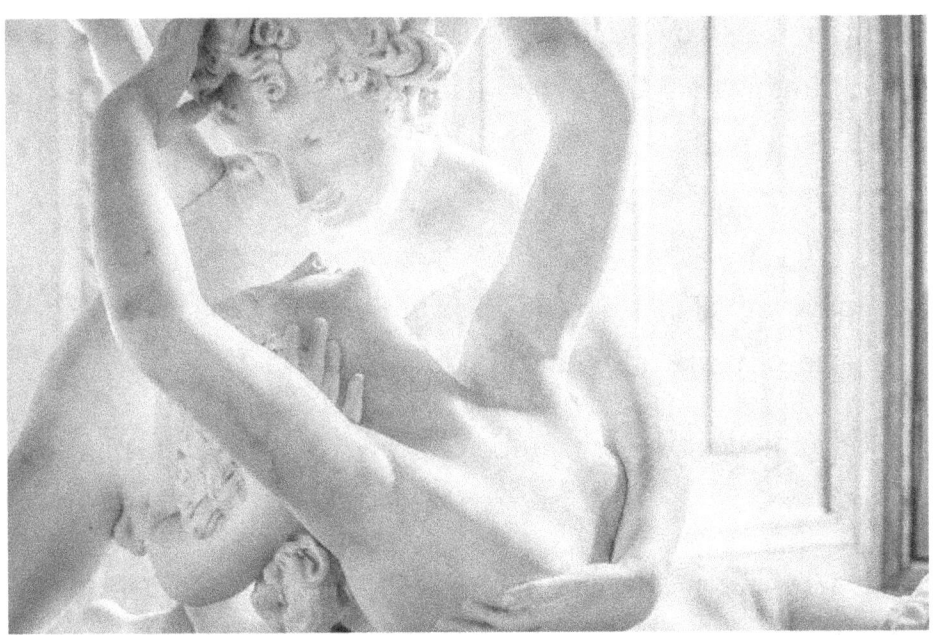

Soaps have different types, they vary in color, scent and the ingredients found on it. These soaps have their own uses and purpose. Like for example, detergents, they are obviously used in cleaning clothes and fabrics. Another one is the dishwashing soap, they are used on cleaning the plates and other utensils at our homes. And there are many more types of soaps with a wide range of use.

Different Kinds of Soaps:

I am sure that there are some of you with a curious mind asks a lot of question, especially about the soap you use. That is why you are here, reading this article. Now I will list down the different kinds of soaps, they're using and how they are made.

- *Toilet Soaps*

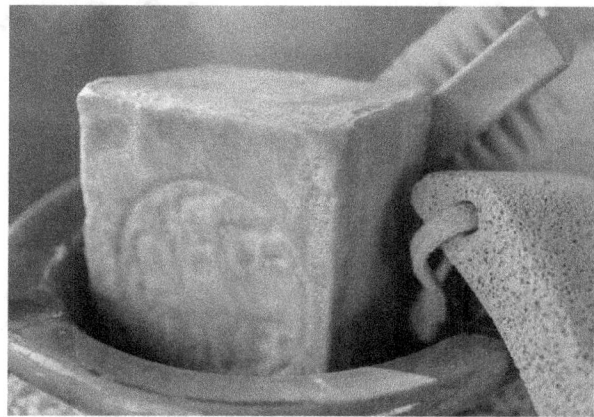

Toilet soaps are the kinds of soaps that are used cosmetically. Toilet soaps are different from bathing soaps, why? Because Totally Fatty Matter or TFM in toilet soaps are large in numbers while on bathing soaps they are low. If the TFM is higher, that only means it is more effective in cleaning. Toilet soaps are divided into three grades.

The first grade contains TFM for about 76%, these soaps are high in quality and they have various colors and scents. The second grade contains TFM for about 70%, these soaps are often smooth and they are commonly white in color. The third grade contains TFM for about 60%, these soaps also have smooth texture on it. But they are commonly red in color due to the acidic content they have. Now knowing all about the grades and some knowledge about the toilet soaps, now I'll be listing down its different kinds.

- *Laundry Soaps*

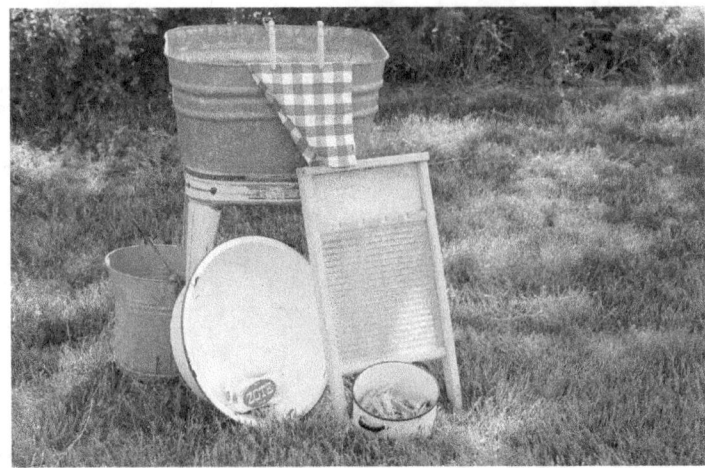

These kind of soaps are the ones we usually see in laundries (well obviously). They can be distinguished as liquid soaps and detergents. The most common ingredient found in a detergent is called surfactant. But you must know that the ingredients every detergent have still varied depending on the brand. There are various ingredients specially used for scents and other characteristics these detergents have. Going back to the surfactant, this ingredient is an active agent.

Surfactants are highly attracted to dirt and water that is why when you use the detergent on laundry, these surfactants attach to the dirt on the clothes and with the help of the water, it pushes the dirt and water upwards to the surface removing the dirt completely from the clothes.

- *Dish Soaps*

Dish soaps are commonly seen as thick liquefied soaps which you need to mix with water in order to use it or sometimes they come in water-based appearance. The ingredients we can commonly see on dish soaps are mint and lemon, why? Is it because they can help easily remove stains from plates and utensils, especially when mixed with warm water.

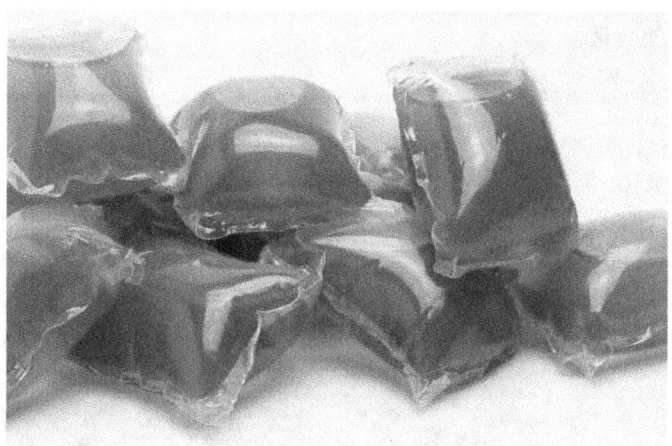

While you scrub the plate with a sponge, this iconic duo (the sponge and the dish soap) will help remove the oils and other unwanted materials from the plates, leaving them on the water's surface ready to be disposed of.

- *Guest Soaps*

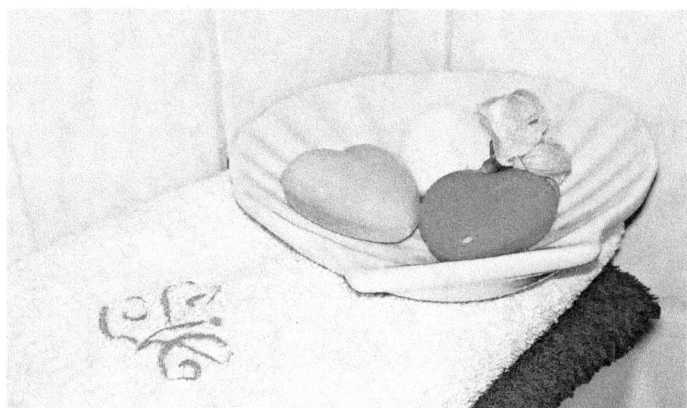

These specific types of soaps are the ones you can see in the hotel rooms. They usually come in small sizes. Imagine them as your standard body cleaning soap. They don't usually have fancy ingredients like essential oils and others. But they do have different scents that you'll like, but remember, bringing them home and stocking them up in place is not recommended. Like said, they are small, that means they usually not last for that long.

- *Beauty Soaps*

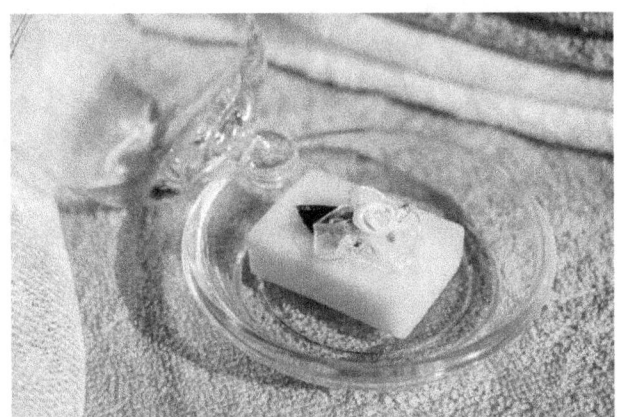

We know that beauty soaps are one of a kind because of the things it offers you, moisturized skin, smooth skin, clearer, and brighter skin and a lot more. There is no doubt that beauty soaps made its way on the top of the kinds of soaps. But be cautious about buying your beauty soaps because not all of them are applicable to your skin. Before buying one, you must know first what skin type you have, then you are good to go. You can choose from the standard bar soaps or the liquefied ones.

- *Medicated Soaps*

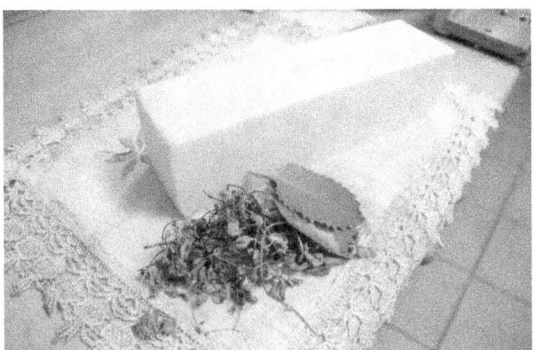

These kinds of soaps are made for one purpose and that is to treat skin diseases and allergies. They help eradicate virus and bacteria from your skin. But the use of medicated soaps is only recommended if the doctor says so.

So all in all, medicated soaps are made with antibacterial ingredients. That is why it is very effective in clearing out your skin off from bacteria and viruses.

- *Novelty Soaps*

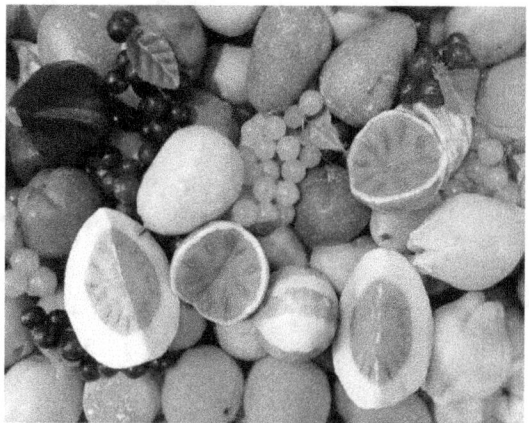

Novelty soaps, they are not your typical soap that cleanses off the germs away. Novelty soap is the kind of soap that is commonly known because of its creative and artistic way of creation. These lovely soaps are best used as gifts for special events like weddings and anniversaries. They are commonly handmade and stands out because of their very soothing fragrance. Well, they may not be your typical soaps, but they can be handy in travels due to their small sizes.

- *Non-Toilet Soaps*

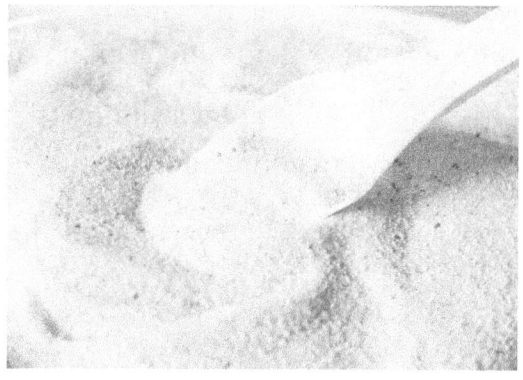

This is the second kind of soap. Well, they are called non-toilet soaps because they are used in heavy cleaning. They are used for removing large amounts of grease and stains. They are not applicable to human skin because they contain acidic ingredients. They are also used as lubricants.

Forms of Soaps (The most common ones)

Of course, if there are different kinds of soap, there will be different forms of it. It may be your standard solid soap or the liquefied ones. So for more information about soaps, I'll be listing down the different forms of soap, the common ones.

Bath Soaps

They appear different from the ones you use in cleaning your whole body while taking a bath and the ones you use just for your face. Bath soaps are generally known for its purpose on making the skin smooth and clean. They can come in bar soaps and sometimes in liquid gels.

Liquid Soaps

The ones we use to buy whenever a bar soap is not available. Liquid soaps are both effective on the whole body and the hands. Also, they are used for the laundry and dishes, one example is the dishwashing liquid.

Liquid soaps have different ingredients or cleaning agents, these depend on the surface they'll be applied on to. The thing that makes liquid soaps stand out from others is that they last longer and easy to bring when going on a travel.

Another thing about liquid soap is that some of them are made of milk, yep you heard that right. These milk soaps are essential for nourishing the skin and making it moisturized and healthy. There are milk soaps used for babies, they are made from goat's milk because goat's milk doesn't contain any harmful elements that can cause irritation on the babies' skin unlike the ones made from artificial materials.

Soaps that gives out good fragrance like the peppermint soap, vanilla soap, seaweed soap and a lot more. These fragrant soaps contain oils that can be found on plants and herbs. These soaps are natural and good for the skin. But apart from others, there are also soaps made out of expensive ingredients or somewhat we can call luxurious. One example are the chocolate soaps (sounds sweet right?), these soaps are made out of cocoa and they can help maintain your skin moisturized.

Bar Soaps

This is the general term for all soap out there (of course I meant for those solid ones and not the liquid versions of them). Bar soaps can be beauty soaps, novelty, laundry or even medicated soaps.

Handmade Soaps

These kind of soaps are by far the safest, why? They are handmade which means they are naturally made, no chemicals added. They are safe for the skin, and what makes these soaps unique is the variety of combinations you can have to create a natural soap.Now you have almost all the knowledge about soaps. So what's next? I bet that you are thinking of creating your own, especially the handmade ones are the safest types right? Don't worry, I got you. I'll be listing down the different methods on how to make soap right at your own home. So what are we waiting for? Let's dive in through this.

Starting with the first method, this is called the "Cold Process Method" (did that just rhyme?). This method is approved and the original one in making soap. So, to start this method, all you need to do is melt down the soft and hard oils together. Then blend it with the lye solution.

But this lye solution and oil solution must be mixed together and melted down with the same temperature, around 90 degrees F. Right after you mixed the two solutions, you need to blend them. This time it is already up to you if you're going to use a blender or you'll blend it manually with a whisk. When properly blended, you can already transfer the mixture into a soap mold. Then you need to cool it down on your fridge for about 4 to 6 weeks before you can put it in action.

The second method is the "Hot Process Method". In this method, the solidification of the soap is much faster, that is why many soap makers really like this method of soap making. To start this method, you're going to melt the oils and mix them with the lye solution. You're going to mix these two mixtures until they become very thick. Then after that, you can pour down the mixture on a soap mold then allow it to cool. When already cooled, you can now use it as a normal soap.

For the third method, it is called the "Room Temperature Method".In this method, all you need to do is gather the hard oils in one container and from there you're going to pour down the hot lye solution. After pouring it, you must stir it gently until the hard oils melt. When the hard oils melt fully, you can now put the soft oils and then blend it all together to form a thick mixture. After creating this mixture, you can now pour it down on a soap mold. Then set it aside for about 4 to 6 weeks like the cold process method before you can use it.

The fourth method is called the "Oven Process Method". This method is actually a general one from the previous three methods. When you are going to use this on the room temperature and cold process methods.

You're going to start on the part where the soap is thick and already poured down on the soap mold, from there you will cook it on the oven for about 150 to 170 degrees F until it becomes gel-like in structure. This method depends on you, some will put the soap molded on the hot oven then turn it off and leave it overnight. And others will cook it for several others. On the other hand, for the hot process method, the oven will be used as the heating device to melt the soap until it becomes thick enough to be poured down on a soap mold.

For the fifth method, it is called the "Whipped Soap Bar Method". This method is quite unique, it doesn't require any heat in order to melt the oils. What you need to do is chill the lye. A soap created using this method has high amounts of hard oils and a few liquid oils. The hard oils in this method are whipped until it becomes thick and soft then the liquid oils will be poured down and blended in. You are going to stir it again and again until it becomes soft and thick like the first mixture.

After achieving this texture, you can now put it in a soap mold then set aside, wait for about 4 to 6 weeks then you're good to go with your homemade soap. The sixth method is called the "Melt and Pour Soap". This method is kinda easy, wait no, actually it is the easiest one because it does not require you to melt down lye solutions and other stuff because it is already premade for you.

What you need to do is just melt this premade lye solution then add your preferred scent and color then pour it right into the soap mold, like the other methods, set aside for weeks then you can use the soap you've just made.

The seventh method is the "Whipped Cream Soap". In this method, you are not making a standard solid soap, but a soap that is soft like whipped cream! This method uses potassium hydroxide and sodium hydroxide and the way to do this one is kind of complicated compared with the other methods listed here. So making this cool soap can take a lot of time and effort.

The eighth method is called the "Glycerin Soap or Transparent Soap". Hence the name, these soaps are transparent. In making a transparent soap, you need to use the hot process method but a little different, when the process reaches on the point of the soap being thick enough, the alcohol and glycerin are now added in order for the soap base to be dissolved.

When the base already melted, on the glycerin solution, there is a sugar solution added in order to help for the transparency of the soap. At this point, you can now add the scent and color of your choice on the mixture. Stir them gently then right after, you can put it now on the soap mold and set it aside for about 4 weeks then you can use your transparent soap. Keep in mind that this step is not that easy because, in some countries, they require you to have this special license in order to buy the alcohol needed for your transparent soap.

For the ninth and last method, it is called the "Liquid Soap Making". Well, in this method, you are making a liquefied soap and this method is the same as the transparent method the only difference is that you don't use sodium hydroxide but you use potassium hydroxide(keep in mind that potassium hydroxide is the main ingredient when making a soft soap or liquid soap).

There are two methods on making liquid soap, they are the alcohol lye method and the paste method. The paste method uses the hot process method until it comes on the procedure's stage of thickening, from there the mixture will be diluted and neutralized then sequestered for weeks.

For the alcohol method, the oils are mixed up with the lye solution, then the alcohol is added then the mixture will be brought to trace. Then right after, the soap will be boiled for hours the same as the paste method, will be diluted and neutralized then sequestered for weeks. To make the most of this method, you should familiarize yourself first with the hot and cold process method.

Chapter 2 – Soap Recipes For Smoother Skin

Ever see a whitening soap or a soap that can make your skin smoother in the mall but you can't afford it? But do you know that you can make these soaps right in your home? Yes, that is right! With the right ingredients, you can make these soaps in no time. They all have the same quality and the best part? The one you make in your home is a lot safer than the commercial ones because of the natural ingredients you'll be using.

Grapefruit Mint Poppy Seed Soap

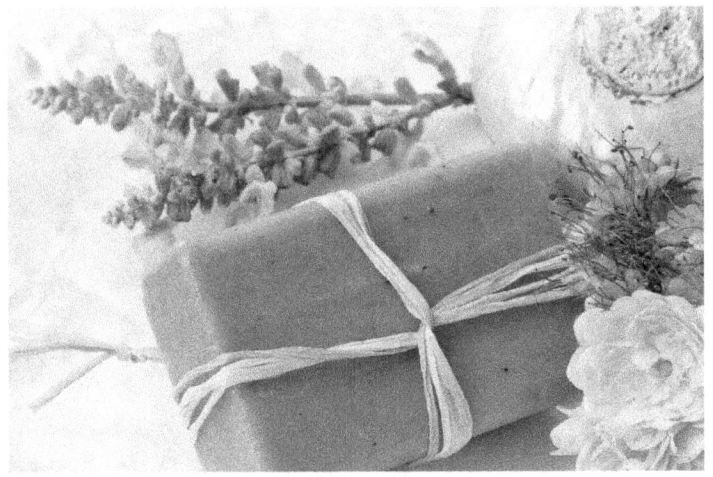

The ingredients you need:

10 oz. <u>goat's milk melt-and-pour soap base</u>
1 grapefruit
1 tbsp. poppy seeds
10 drops of <u>grapefruit essential oil</u>
4 drops of <u>peppermint essential oil</u>

Procedure:

1. Get your goat milk soap base then cut it into cubes.
2. Scrape the grapefruit you have then prepare the poppy seeds.
3. Set your microwave in a standard heating mode or prepare your stove for boiling then melt the soap on either of the two.
4. While it melts, stir it gently. Be careful not to burn the soap.
5. When the soap is already melted, put it in a container where it can fit exactly, then add the grapefruit you've just scraped, the poppy seeds and the oils.
6. Stir the mixture you've just made.
7. Then next is, pour the melted soap mixture on the soap mold then set aside until it gets hard. It will usually take about 2 to 3 hours before it completely hardens.
8. When it is hard already, you can pop them out from the mold and use them (you can also prepare them as gifts).

Aloe Vera Soap

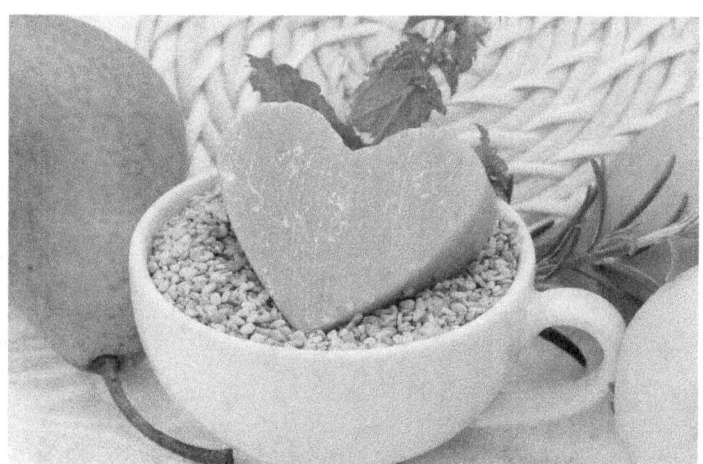

The ingredients you need:

14.9 oz. <u>coconut oil</u>

13.4 oz. <u>olive oil</u>

10.5 oz. <u>lard</u>

2.5 oz. <u>shea butter</u>

9.6 oz. g <u>aloe gel</u> and water purée

6.7 oz. <u>lye (NaOH)</u>

9.9 oz. water

Procedure:

1. On a bowl or any container of your choice, pour the water and add the lye.
2. On a stove or a microwave oven, heat up and melt the oils.
3. When the oil melts, add the lye mixture to the melted oil.
4. Right after adding the lye mixture, add the aloe gel.
5. Mix them well until the mixture becomes thick enough.
6. Pour the mixture on a soap mold and set aside for about a day or two.
7. When it hardens already, you can now use it.

Vanilla Citrus Soap

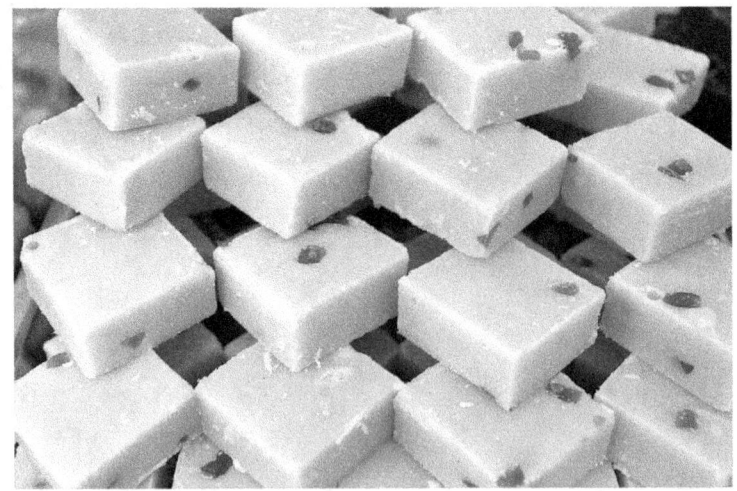

The ingredients you need:

6 small cubes of melt & pour soap base

Vanilla essential oil or extract

Orange peel

Poppy seeds

Silicone Molds

Procedure:

1. Meltdown the small cubes of your soap base in a microwave (be sure to put it on a microwavable bowl).
2. While the soap base on the process of melting, zest the orange peel.
3. When the soap is already melted, remove it from the microwave and prepare it for pouring in the mold.
4. On a bowl, pour down the melted soap base and then add the orange zest, poppy seeds, and the vanilla oil, stir them gently.
5. When they are already mixed up well, carefully pour the mixture on the silicone molds.
6. Set aside for about 2 hours.
7. When they are already hard, you can pop them off from the silicone mold and now ready for use.

Chapter 3 – DIY Germicidal Soap Recipes

A bit more conscious about the soap you use? Of course, the first thing that comes to mind is to buy a soap that can protect you from certain viruses and bacteria that can cause skin allergies. But, like the most soaps, you can make your own antibacterial soap right in your home!

Shea Butter with Coconut Milk Soap

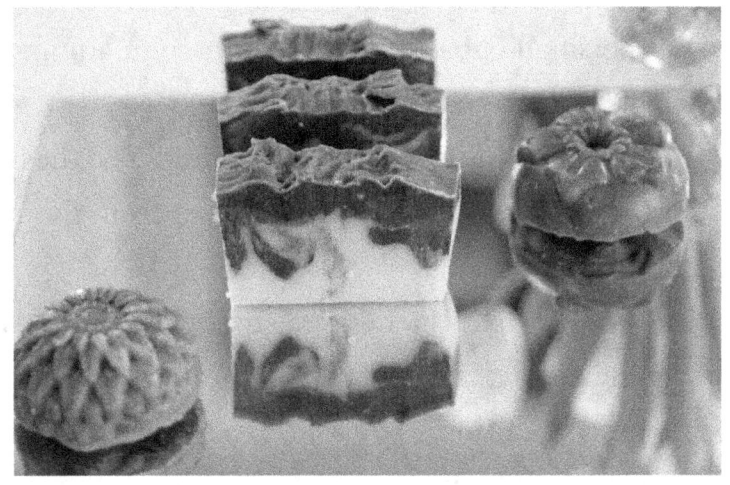

The ingredients you need:

Shea Butter -135 gr.

Coconut Oil -6.35 oz.

Olive Oil -12.7 oz.

Castor Oil - 3.175 oz.

Palm Oil- 4.8 oz.

Distilled Water -7.05 oz.

Coconut Milk -3.42 oz.

Lye -4.34 oz.

Calendula Flower Petals

Procedure:

1. On a pan, warm up the coconut milk and then set it aside.
2. Follow the standard soap making method on making your soap batter (mix the water and lye).
3. Finely mince the Calendula flower petals.
4. Make a thin trace from this soap batter mixture. Then right after add the coconut milk.
5. Stir the mixture gently until it reaches a medium trace.
6. Get your soap mold and then pour down ¾ of the soap batter.
7. On the remaining soap batter, add the Calendula flower petals and stir it well.
8. Then add the remaining soap batter on the mold.
9. Set it aside for about a week until it gets hard.
10. Once hard, you can now pop it off from the soap mold and use it.

Olive Oil Soap

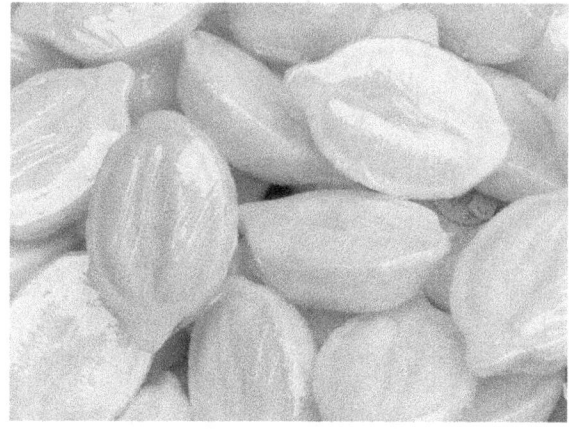

The ingredients you need:

Coconut Oil - 6.35 oz.

Infused Olive Oil - 19.05 oz.

Palm Oil - 6.35 oz.

Distilled Water - 11.5 oz.

Lye - 4.27 oz.

Dried chamomile and calendula

Procedure:

1. To start off in making this antibacterial soap, mix the olive oil and the dried calendula and chamomile.
2. Using a pot, put it on low heat for an hour then right after, set aside and leave overnight.
3. After setting it aside, drain the extract leaving the solid materials.
4. Make the soap mixture by mixing the water and lye.
5. Melt the soap mixture and then add the olive oil mixture on it.
6. When the soap mixture comes into a thin trace, you can now pour it into the soap mold.
7. Set aside for about 4 to 6 weeks and then you can use the soap right after.

Chapter 4 – Colorful Soap Recipes

One thing that makes soap popular in the market is because of its artistic designs. Some soaps are made for decorations, these soaps are called "Novelty Soaps". By having this cool and unique designs on the soap, take note that they are not as effective as an original soap. They can clean but not that much. But don't worry, if you are an artist like me, then let's dive right into making these colorful and unique soaps.

Swirly Soap

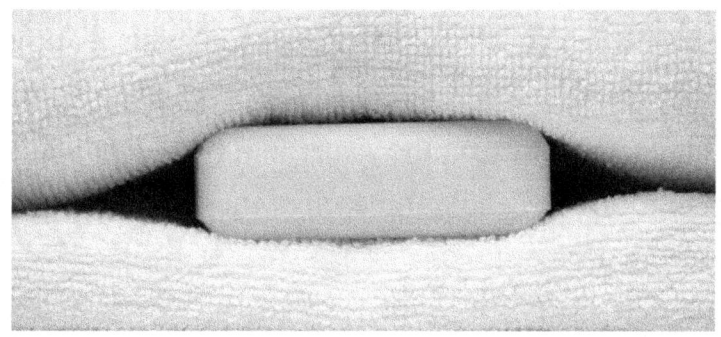

The ingredients you need:

Coconut Oil - 9.52 oz.

Olive Oil - 12.7 oz.

Castor Oil - 1.59 oz.

Palm Oil- 7.94 oz.

Distilled Water - 12.06 oz.

Lye - 129.15 gr.

Cocoa Powder - 1/4 Tsp.

Black Oxide - 1/4 Tsp.

Yellow Oxide - 1/4 Tsp.

White Mica - 1 1/4 Tsp.

Procedure:

1. By doing this recipe, you need to follow the "Room Temperature Method" recently discussed.
2. Mix the oils, water, and the lye to make the soap mixture.
3. Mix the soap mixture on a warm heat until it reaches a thin trace.
4. After reaching a thin trace, get a soap mold with four molds on it (you're going to use these four spaces for the colors).
5. Pour the soup mixture on the soap mold (equally divided on the four molds).
6. One by one, add each color on each of the four molds.
7. Mix them gently.
8. Grab another soap mold.
9. On the other soap mold, drizzle down one soap color then add the other three (drizzle it on a swirling pattern).
10. When they are all mixed up and swirled, you can now set aside the soap to make it hard.
11. Once the soap hardens, you can now pop it off from the soap mold and use it, or gift wrap it and use it as a gift for a friend or relative on a special event.

Coffee Soap

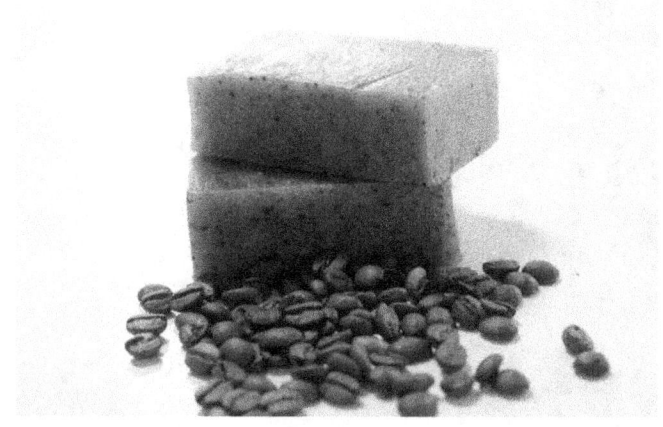

The ingredients you need:

Shea Butter - 135 gr.

Coconut Oil - 7.9 oz.

Olive Oil - 11.1 oz.

Castor Oil - 3.18 oz.

Palm Oil - 4.76 oz.

Distilled Water - 324 gr.

Lye - 125.25 gr.

Essential Oils of Ginger - 1/2 tsp.

Essential Oils of Cinnamon - 1/2 tsp.

Essential Oils of Clove - 1/2 Tsp.

Essential Oils of Patchouli- 1/2 Tsp.

Essential Oils of Sweet Orange - 6 Tsp.

Finely Ground Oatmeal - 2 Tbsp.

Cocoa Powder - 1 tsp.

Finely ground coffee - 1 Tbsp.

Confectioners' Sugar - 1 tsp.

Orris Root Powder - 1 tsp.

Procedure:

1. Prepare the oils, the water and the lye. On this part of the procedure, it is up to you on what soap making method you are going to use.
2. Once the soap mixture is created. Stir it until it reaches a thin trace.
3. After reaching a thin trace, pour ¼ of the soap mixture into the soap mold.
4. Right there, add the cocoa powder, ground coffee, Orris root powder, ground oatmeal and sugar, mix them well.
5. Pour down all the essential oils on the mixture and mix them quickly.
6. Then you can now set it aside.
7. When it is hard already, you can now use it or make it as a gift for someone special.

Chapter 5 – Creative Multipurpose Soap Recipes

The large variety of soaps have their own purpose. But what if you can have a soap that is antibacterial and at the same time a beauty soap? Isn't that convenient for you? But sadly, some of these high-quality multipurpose soaps are expensive in the market but don't you worry, I'll be helping you on making your own multipurpose soap right in your own home. So what are you waiting for? Let's start with the first multipurpose soap recipe.

Anise Soap

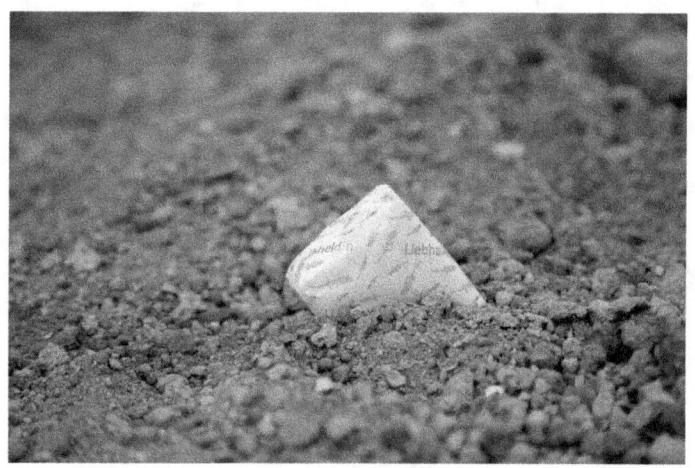

The ingredients you need:

Shea Butter - 45 gr.

Coconut Oil - 7.937 oz.

Olive Oil - 11.11 oz.

Castor Oil - 1.587 oz.

Palm Oil - 9.524 oz.

Distilled Water - 6.31 oz.

Coconut Milk - 3.53 oz.

Lye - 127.05 gr.

Essential Oils of Anise - 1/2 Tsp.

Essential Oils of Sweet Fennel - 1/2 Tsp.

Essential Oils of Sweet Orange - 2 Tsp.

Essential Oils of Cinnamon - 1/4 tsp.

Essential Oils of Clove Bud - 1/4 Tsp.

Essential Oils of Nutmeg - 1/4 tsp.

Rose Fragrance Oil - 4 Tsp.

White Mica - 1 Tsp.

Black Oxide - 1/2 Tsp.

Orris Root Powder - 1 Tsp.

Procedure:

1. In this soap recipe, it is also up to you on what soap making method you are going to use.
2. Once you've picked your preferred soap making method, start by mixing the shea butter, coconut oil, olive oil, palm oil, castor oil, water, and the lye on a bowl or a container where they can all fit.
3. When already mixed, you've just made your soap mixture.
4. Continue mixing the mixture until it comes into a thin trace.
5. When it reaches the thin trace, add the coconut milk, white mica, Orris root powder, the rose fragrance scent, and the black oxide.
6. Stir the mixture well until it reaches a medium trace.

7. When already on medium trace, you can now pour down the mixture on the soap mold.

8. Finish the procedure based on the soap making method you've chosen.

Matcha Soap

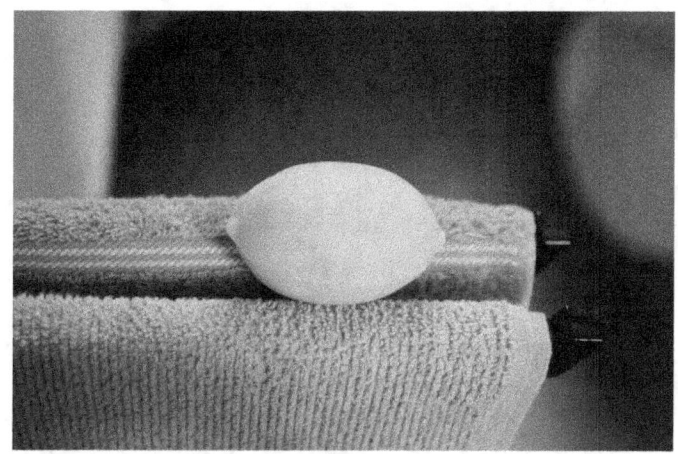

The ingredients you need:

1 pound melt & pour glycerin soap

2 tbsp. matcha powder

3/4 tsp. lemon essential oil

Soap Mold

Procedure:

1. Slice the 1 pound melt and pour the soap into small pieces and put them in a microwavable bowl.

2. Set the microwave to high heat and then put the bowl with the soap inside.

3. Let it sit there for about 30 seconds.

4. After that, get the bowl and stir it gently then put it back on the microwave for about 15 seconds or 20 seconds.
5. After that, get the bowl out of the microwave and then stir again.
6. Repeat step 4 and 5 until the soap melts completely.
7. When the soap already melts, get it out of the microwave and then add the matcha powder and the lemon essential oil. Stir well.
8. Now the soap is ready to be poured down on the soap mold.
9. After putting it on the soap mold, you can now let it sit for about a week before you can use it.

Cream Soap

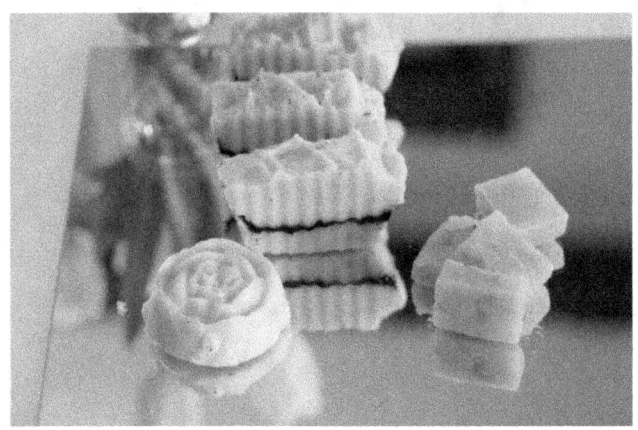

The ingredients you need:

1 bar soap

4-6 cups water

1 tsp. Glycerin

2 cups vegetable shortening

1 cup of coconut oil

10-15 drops essential oils (optional)

Procedure:

1. Start by shredding the bar of soap, after shredding it, set the soap aside.
2. Prepare your stove to medium heat and then on a pot, put the shredded soap and add 4 cups of water. Let it sit on medium heat for about 30 minutes.
3. After the 30 minutes time interval, add the glycerin on the melted soap, stir it well.
4. Pour down the mixture of the soap and glycerin on Styrofoam cups and let it cool.
5. You'll notice that the soap will slowly turn thick.
6. Put the soap on a bowl and let it cool again.
7. As the soap is in the process of cooling down, start making the whip.
8. Grab a large bowl, and there, add the coconut oil and the vegetable shortening.
9. Mix these two ingredients until it becomes thick.
10. When it becomes thick already, you can now add the cooled down soap.
11. Whip the soap and the mixture until it turns into a whipped cream texture.
12. Add the optional essential oil then you're good to go.

Peppermint Soap

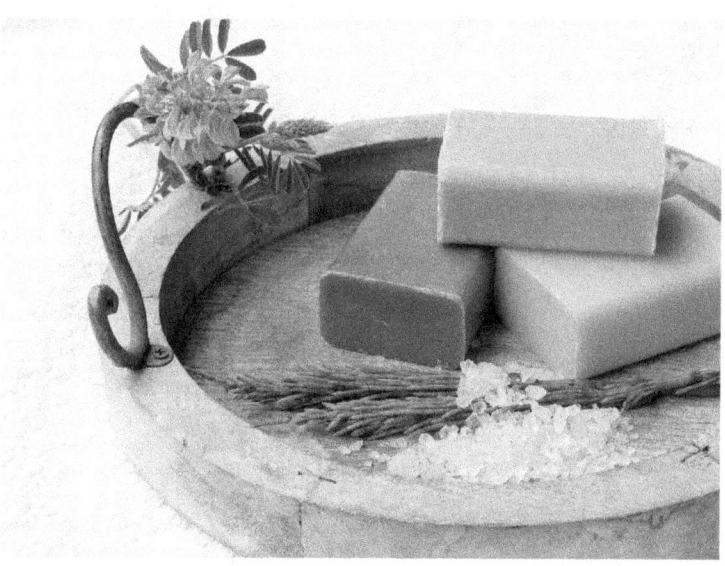

The ingredients you need:

2 lbs. _Shea butter melt and pour soap_

Peppermint Oil

1 box Crushed Candy Canes

Rubbing Alcohol in a spray bottle

Soap Mold

Procedure:

1. On a pot, melt down the shea butter and pour soap for about an hour.
2. When the shea butter and the soap already melt, add about 10 to 12 drops of peppermint oil, mix well.
3. Prepare the soap mold, spray it with rubbing alcohol so that bubbles from the soap will not be created.
4. Now pour the melted soap on the soap mold then add the crushed candy canes on the top.
5. The next thing to do is wrap the soap and let it sit for about 2 hours so that it will not dry out while in the process of hardening.
6. When the soap is already hard, you can now use it or wrap it as a gift.

Conclusion

So if you want to take your life to the next level and make something new out of your creativity then you can make use of the soap recipes that we have discussed. Once you mastered this lovely soap making craft, you can modify the ingredients and shapes according to your own preferences.

I hope that you have learned a lot from this book and I am looking forward to your growth no matter what plan do you have in your new craft whether you will just use it for your own personal use or make it as a business it's up for you to decide.

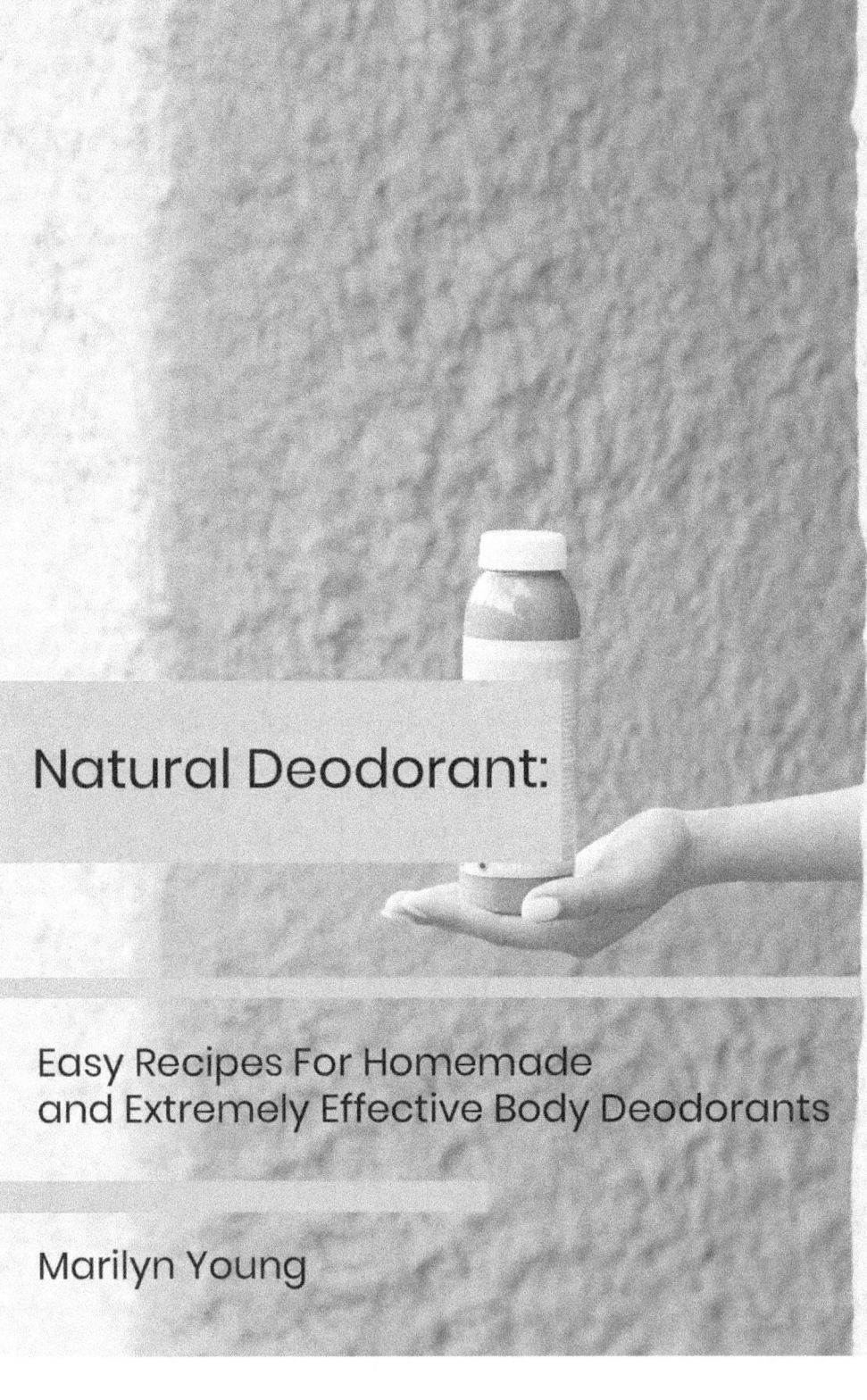

Natural Deodorant:

Easy Recipes For Homemade and Extremely Effective Body Deodorants

Marilyn Young

Natural Deodorant:

Easy Recipes For Homemade and Extremely Effective Body Deodorants

Introduction:

Modern girls find it difficult to imagine the morning without the use of the favorite deodorant. But how often do we consider the fact that the harm from this product is bigger than benefit? The debate about the safety of antiperspirants has been going on almost since they appeared on the shelves of pharmacies. The detrimental effect of these cosmetics is due to the presence of aluminum and zinc.

Getting on the skin, antiperspirant forms a special film. Its task is to block the sweat glands, and, therefore, to prevent the occurrence of an unpleasant odor. But not everything is so simple. Sweating is a natural property of the human body. With its help, toxic substances are removed and the body temperature is maintained. Simply put, the use of antiperspirant interferes with natural cleansing.

If you ask doctors, you will suddenly know the shocking truth. Particularly, the use of antiperspirants is one of the causes of breast cancer. This is due to the action of parabens - preservatives, commonly used in the cosmetic industry. The carcinogenicity of these substances is still questionable, but many women are already switching to natural self-care products. What is to replace the antiperspirant from the store? The best option is a tool made with your own hands.

Which benefits does home-made deodorant have?

Firstly, they do not contain any health risks. Consider the difference between antiperspirant and deodorant. Many believe that this is the same thing but there are significant differences in the operation of these means. For instance, the antiperspirant clogs the glands and blocks sweating

Deodorant, in turn, destroys microorganisms that live in the ducts of sweat glands and cause an unpleasant smell. At the same time the process of sweating is preserved, and harmful substances do not linger in the body. Deodorants are difficult to find in stores, but can be made from scrap materials.

As well, such recipes of homemade deodorants are approved by several generations. The beneficial properties of soda, citrus essential oils and cocoa were successfully used long before the mass production of cosmetics. Finally, in contrast to the "biting" prices of cosmetics of famous brands, the cost of the components of home deodorant will delight you. Ingredients for such a tool can be found in the kitchen or bought at a nearby supermarket.

Chapter 1 – Why people all over the world opt for natural deodorants

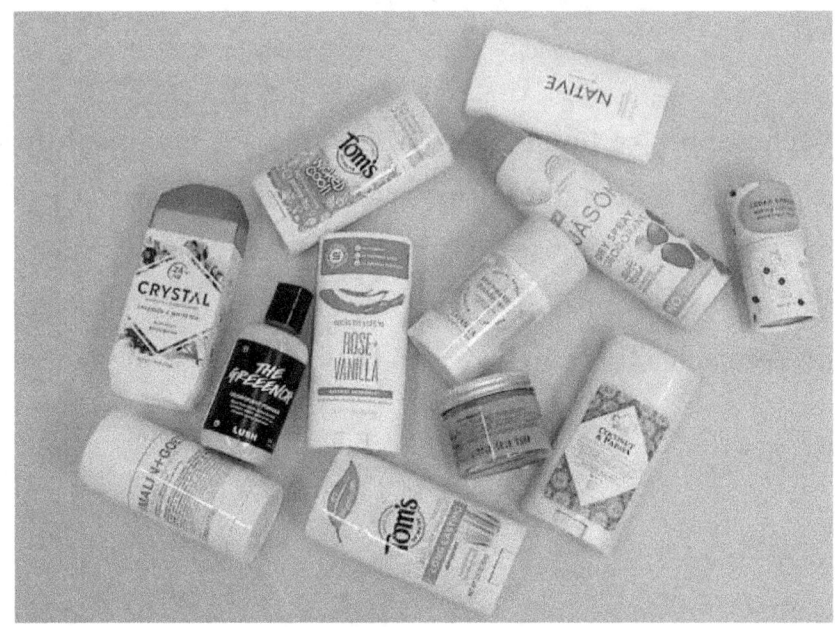

Today more and more people all around the world are making their choice in favor of natural deodorants. Not only do they reject from the chemical analogues but also dedicate their time to creation of deodorants on their own.

Sweating is a natural process that allows the body to maintain a constant temperature, and it helps us we feel quite comfortable. But if a person sweats intensely, it affects the quality of his life badly. Such a situation is getting abnormal, that's why people can speak about hyperhidrosis, mean, excessive sweating. The same applies to the strong smell of sweat, a condition called bromidrosis. Everyone tries to cope with this problem in different ways, but often the chosen means are ineffective and sometimes even harmful. In most cases, excessive sweating is just a feature of the body.

If you are actively sweating from adolescence or at least 25 years old, then this is the case. An unpleasant odor occurs due to the fact that bacteria recycle compounds contained in sweat and skin, and as a result, bad-smelling substances such as ammonia are formed. It can be especially noticeable among people with too much sweat - the bacteria in these favorable conditions become larger and the scale of production of odorous substances increases. That is, bromidrosis and hyperhidrosis are often related phenomena.

Although sometimes it may be that a person has too many specific sweat glands (apocrine), which secrete not a liquid, but a fatty substance (mostly it happens when a person is nervous). Because of that, smell appears. If excessive sweating appears after the person is over 25 years old, it can be the cause of some disease or medication, especially if a person is sweating at night or suddenly lost weight. There is a great deal of diseases and conditions leading to hyperhidrosis, from menopause to tuberculosis.

Therefore, it is better not to deal with the symptoms, but go to the doctor who will find the cause. There is absolutely no need to hesitate whether it is worth visiting a specialist if there is dizziness, chest pain or nausea. There are also quite a lot of medications for which a person begins to sweat more intensively (among them, for example, nitroglycerin and some antidepressants), but you shouldn't stop them without a doctor.

An unpleasant smell of sweat from the whole body, and not from the legs or armpits, can also be a sign of the disease, but usually in this case there are other severe symptoms. More often the case is in the diet - garlic, onion, curry and alcohol can affect the smell of sweat. Antiperspirants and deodorants are the next things a doctor will recommend after basic hygiene practices.

Deodorants should mask the smell of sweat, that is, one smell should interrupt the other. They also often contain alcohol, which results in the formation of an acidic environment on the skin that is uncomfortable for bacteria. The effectiveness of this approach is not very large, and deodorants can save only in the easiest cases.

Antiperspirants work because aluminum salts (usually aluminum chloride, also aluminum chloride hexahydrate) clog pores from which sweat comes out. Theoretically, even the most common antiperspirants (with a low concentration of aluminum salts) can cause swelling and irritation of the skin, but in practice this is quite rare.

Do not be afraid of the fact that over time there will be addiction to antiperspirants and they will have to be applied more often. Antiperspirants need to be used correctly. Ordinary antiperspirants are recommended to be applied after a shower on dry skin. However, right after this, you should not sweat for the remedy to work. Therefore, the American Academy of Dermatology generally advises the use of antiperspirants before bedtime.

Antiperspirants, in which the concentration of aluminum chloride is above 6%, are also recommended to be applied to clean, dry skin at bedtime. Because of numerous problems connected to the deodorants and antiperspirants which we have bought in the shops, nowadays more and more people tend to make this product at home.

We will tell you how to do it with the least efforts.

Chapter 2 – The most harmful ingredients which you never need in deodorants

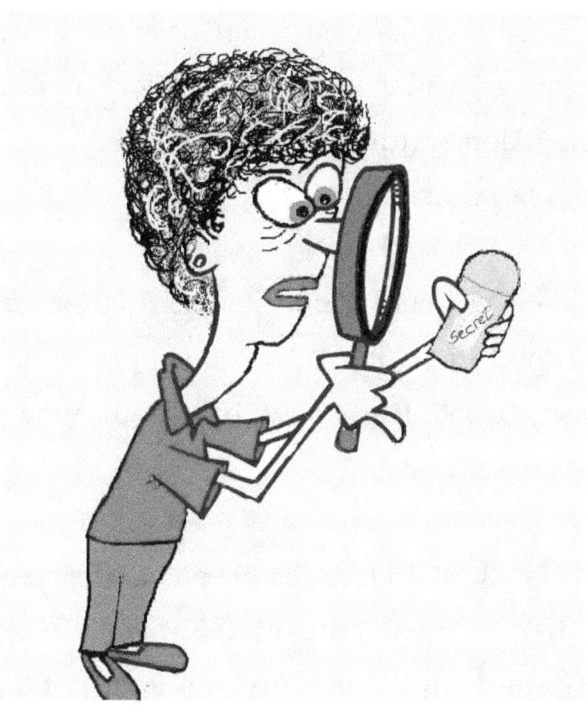

Why do you need a substitute for deodorant? Now the market proposes a lot of deodorants of different shapes, smell and composition. However, they also contain hazardous substances, such as aluminum. We use deodorant every day, rubbing it into the skin. In such a way aluminum penetrates the body, causing hormonal disruptions, premature aging, Alzheimer's disease and even cancer. Sometimes it may not contain aluminum, but it is often replaced by other chemicals.

Doctors have proven that sweat is the usual moisture that our glands secrete, and it does not smell. The smell comes from bacteria that are actively developing in a humid environment, and it may depend on gender, diet, drugs, and other factors. Vegetarians claim that the rejection of animal food helps to get rid of the unpleasant smell of sweat.

If you care about your health but don't believe how important natural deodorants are, pay attention to the chemical components in your product. It can be aluminum as it clogs the sweat glands, after which swelling may occur.

The next harmful component is paraben used as preservatives. This substance causes allergies, in severe cases, asphyxiation. Next, triclosan is considered as the most dangerous "killer" of bacteria. Along with the bacteria that cause smell, it destroys the beneficial protective microflora of the skin.

Perhaps, you have never heard about it, but triclosan is banned for use in cosmetics in America and Europe. Then, it comes down to deodorants. Synthetic fragrances give deodorants a pleasant smell. However, it quickly disappears, and the perfumes have time to harm health.

After that, propylene glycol is the substance is antibacterial, but causes problems with the liver and kidneys. In the United States and Europe, its use is prohibited. Finally, alcohol that has a bactericidal effect may cause dryness and irritation. Indeed, only because of our laziness and lack of desire to create a new product hand-made, we push ourselves in the depth of harmful elements which poison our bodies inside.

So, which things are necessary for beautiful look, amazing smell, and good health condition?

Chapter 3 – The best components to include in natural deodorants

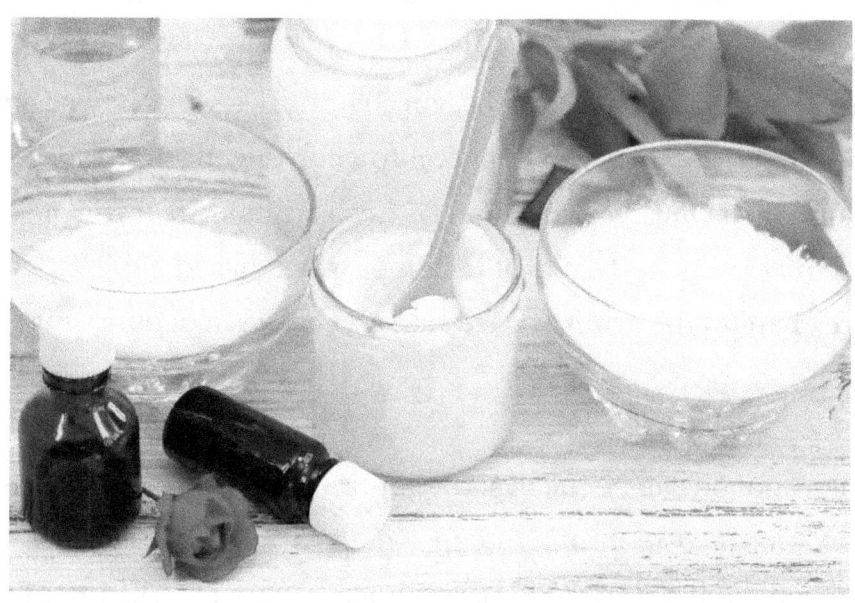

Natural deodorants substitutes contain natural ingredients: *essential oils, coconut oil, natural starch, and alum stone.*The problem of unpleasant smell was tried to be solved even before the invention of deodorants. By the way, in clothes from natural fabrics it is less noticeable. Try using a natural substitute for deodorants, and you will see the result immediately! Not only will you like the smell, but also you are about to feel healthier.

Soda is the most popular "wrestler" with a smell. Soda will not stop sweating, but at the same time, won't allow bacteria to multiply. Soda can be used in different forms; particularly, it might be dry as a powder. Then, it is likely to bring a perfect solution in warm water for rinsing or a mixture with starch, to reduce the "moisture". In such a powder for the smell, you can add a few drops of essential oils.Regular baking soda can be diluted in water and wiped with an armpit cotton pad. It does not relieve sweat, but there is no smell. On very hot days, the procedure should be repeated. However, one factor should be taken in consideration.

If you have very sensitive skin, soda can overdry it. Thus, everything is good when it is measured. In case you are into different sophisticated tastes, you choice has to turn next to essential oils. They are extremely pleasant, and have smoothing and healing effect on the skin and total emotional state. Oil of lavender, fir, pine, tea tree, geranium, wormwood, rosemary, fennel, clove, orange tree, eucalyptus, bergamot, cedar and thyme have antiseptic properties.It is a good idea to apply oil to your finger and rub into areas where there is an unpleasant smell.Once you are fond of fresh fruits or feel thirsty during the hot days, you might rub into the skin the sap of lemon or water-based apple cider vinegar. The aim of this substance changes the acidity of the skin and causes a deodorizing effect.

As well, coconut oil can be the basis of natural deodorant. If you want to make it natural, add *to 5 teaspoons of coconut oil 1/4 cup soda, 1/4 cup starch and essential oils.* First mix the dry ingredients (starch and soda), and then coconut oil. If the oil is too thick, heat it in a microwave or in a water bath. You can also add wax. The mixture is placed in a jar or in a package from under the deodorant and use as an ordinary deodorant. Keep better in the refrigerator. Herbs are also necessary. Infusions of calamus, willow bark, wormwood, thyme, chamomile, coriander are made in cold water, and not boiled.

If you have desire to use oak bark, you are highly likely to prepare a decoction. It might be done in the following way: take 1 tablespoon of crushed bark in a glass of water. Afterwards, wet the cotton pad in the broth and wipe the body. As a substitute for deodorant, burnt alum (aluminum potassium alum) is widely used, but it is aluminum salts, which adversely affects the brain, causes allergies, and damages the immune system. The most convenient option is a mixture based on oils. Ingredients (essential oils, soda, starch, beeswax) are easy to buy and cook very simply. This deodorant can use a year. After the deodorant has been applied, wait 5 minutes so that there are no marks on the clothes.

Chapter 4 – How to create deodorants from coconut and vanilla?

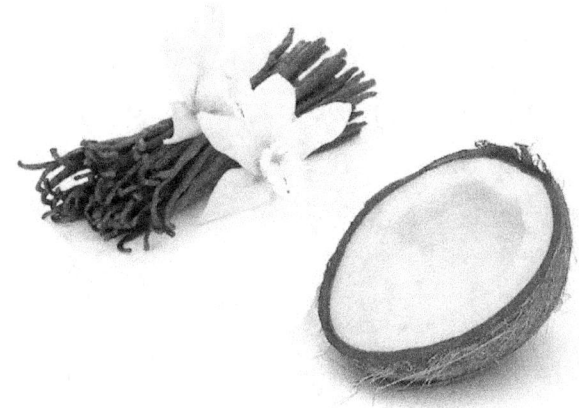

Natural deodorant for the body does not clog pores, does not contain aluminum, lead, parabens. Unfortunately, all these harmful substances are contained in industrial deodorants. They have a peculiarity to accumulate in the body, moreover, it is believed that they can cause breast cancer.

In the modern rhythm of life, many people cannot survive without deodorant, and continue to consciously poison themselves with chemistry to disguise an undesirable smell, this is not the way out. So, you might try to make your own hands a simple, natural and safe for health deodorant. Its production will take not so much time, and all the ingredients that you need, you can easily find on the shelves of shops, pharmacies or on the Internet.

Let's start with two most popular smells of the modern aroma therapy, in particular, coconut oil and vanilla. Firstly, why don't you try **solid natural deodorant with coconut oil**! For that, you need 50 grams of soda. Actually, have you ever heard that baking soda itself is a natural deodorizer?

The next ingredient is 50 grams of corn starch which absorbs, protects and dries the skin. Tea tree essential oil is necessary in the amount of 8-10 drops. However, if desired, you can increase or decrease the amount of essential oil or replace it with another.

Concerning the coconut oil, 2-3 tablespoons will be enough. It is necessary because of ability to soften and moisturize the skin. It is quickly absorbed, and does not leave a fat mark. Also, it serves to impart hardness to deodorant.

When everything is ready, you should follow the next steps:

1. Mix soda with corn starch, add essential oil of tea tree.

2. Next, add coconut oil, which can be pre-melted in a water bath to better mix the ingredients.

3. Put the mixture in the tube from the antiperspirant and put in a cold place for complete solidification.

After a couple of days, the deodorant will become harder.

Application: apply to the skin of the armpits with a thin layer without much effort. This will make your deodorant invisible on the skin and increase its lifespan. For sensitive skin, the amount of corn starch should be increased to 80 g, and soda should be reduced to 30 g.

It is recommended to store in the refrigerator. This deodorant can be prepared in two forms, solid and powdered. Powdered deodorant differs from solid in the absence of coconut oil. They need to gently slap the skin of the armpits.

One more popular thing is beeswax. It might become a good basis for your natural deodorant. Thus, the next recipe is **solid natural deodorant with beeswax**. To prepare it, take 6 grams of beeswax, 24 grams of coconut or palm oil, 24 grams of baking soda, 16 grams of corn or potato starch, and finally 15 drops of essential oils.

Go through this list step by step:

1. 1.Mix well soda and starch.

2. Melt beeswax in a water bath, send coconut oil or palm oil to be heated there.

3. Pour mixed soda with starch into the resulting substance and mix everything.

4. Add essential oils and mix everything thoroughly. Put the mixture in a silicone mold for ice or in a deodorant tube. Put in the fridge until it solidifies.

Due to the presence of beeswax, such a deodorant in the refrigerator is not necessary to store. Essential oils for natural home deodorants can be chosen in accordance to your preferences. Otherwise, you might listen to the advice of those who are experts.For example, you have a wide range to choose from, especially, tea tree, lavender, verbena, rosewood, vanilla, geranium, juniper, nutmeg, pine, spruce, palmarosa, and vetiver. However, once you can boast sensitive skin, you need something different. Well, thank to a huge variety of natural materials, there is nothing easier than choosing the one you need for your skin.

Natural deodorant for sensitive skin is going to be prepared like that. You have to take one tablespoon of corn or potato starch . one tablespoon of baking soda, one tablespoon of beeswas, the same amount of coconut or cedar oil, pour refined shea butter (as well, 1 tsp), add stearic acid at the tip of a knife and put from three to five drops of essential oils.

After the fundamental is ready, do the following actions:

1. Mix soda and starch together.
2. On a water bath, melt the wax, shea butter, coconut oil (cedar)
3. Mix the mixture with soda and starch.
4. Add stearic acid and essential oils.
5. Mix everything thoroughly. Transfer to a container from a deodorant or in a mold.
6. Leave in the refrigerator until full freezing.

Chapter 5 – The best ways to use aloe in natural deodorants

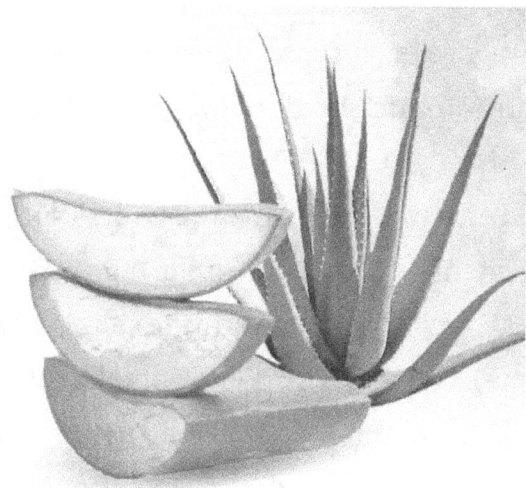

The natural deodorants are based on natural absorbents that take away sweat and odor neutralizing agents. Usually it is clay, soda, essential oils. You can also choose the form of a deodorant, particularly, opt for liquid or solid one. The second most popular component after the coconut is aloe. Especially, it is indispensable once you have decided to **make a solid deodorant**.

To prepare your own smell, you don't need to get a special education of perfumer. Instead, take the following ingredients:

1/4 cup coconut oil
1/4 cup shea butter,
1/4 cup beeswax granules
1 tablespoon glycerin,
1 tablespoon of aloe vera gel,
1 tablespoon of baking soda,
20 drops of essential oil of tea tree or eucalyptus,
20 drops of mint or lavender essential oil.

Melt the beeswax oil in a small saucepan and add glycerin and aloe vera to it. Mix the oil mixture, soda and essential oils in a separate container. Allow the mixture to cool and pour into old deodorant packaging. You can also pour the mixture into silicone molds for cupcakes. As we have already discussed the importance of natural deodorants, it might look like a spray. If you are into such kinds of things, study the benefits of the natural components.

To make **spray deodorant at home**, take one spray bottle, 1/4 cup of strong alcohol, vinegar (actually, it might be unfiltered apple, but you can also use plain white) - 2 teaspoons. Next, don't forget about a pinch of natural salt (as well, it is good idea to choose pink Himalayan or sea one). As well, why don't you take essential oils? Their amount may vary to your taste (for example, you are likely to get a good smell having combined lavender and geranium oil). Generally, it is advised to take 15 drops of each essential oil. Additionally, take one tablespoon of aloe.

The method of preparation includes the following steps:

1. 1)Pour salt in a bottle, add essential oils, aloe vera and pour alcohol and a bite.

2. 2) Shake well. Thus, you have seen how easy it is to prepare it at home. Once we have talked about the usage, after a shower or bath, sprinkle 2-3 times in the right place.

Actually, while making a choice in favor of natural aloe deodorant, you should consider some important facts:

- Give your armpits time to get used to the natural deodorant. The first days of use you probably have to put more. But over time, the glands will change and you will sweat less and the unpleasant smell will disappear.

- When applied to freshly shaved skin, it will pinch!

- Deodorant will not smell of vinegar, but only the essential oils that you add to them. So feel free to combine your favorite smells!

- Using this deodorant you will sweat! What you should do! Sweating is a way to remove toxins from our body, so in no case should we stop it.

- This deodorant does not whiten and does not leave stains on clothes.

As there are a lot of recipes of spray deodorants which you might prepare at home, you can **try another option**. Spray differs in an economic expense, as well, it can be taken with itself in the road.

1. Fill with cold water (250 ml) a couple of tablespoons of dry herbal. Pharmacy chamomile, train, linden have excellent antibacterial action.

2. Bring the infusion to a boil, hold on the fire for 15-20 minutes, cool and strain.

3. Add 2-4 tbsp. tablespoons of baking soda and the same amount of aloe juice.

4. The role of fragrance performs any essential oil - 6-7 drops is enough.

5. Stir the mixture thoroughly, pour into a bottle with a spray. Store in a dry cool place for no more than a week. Before use, be sure to shake the bottle so that there is no sediment.

To make a liquid deodorant at home, mix baking soda and cornstarch and add a few drops of your favorite essential oil, such as lavender. Natural liquid deodorants can also be prepared by mixing the extract of witch hazel, aloe vera juice, mineral water, glycerin and antibacterial essential oils. Alum has been used for personal hygiene for many centuries. Mineral crystals are also used as natural deodorants, since they create an environment in which bacteria cannot multiply. Mineral crystals kill bacteria that cause an unpleasant odor.

Chapter 6 – For those who love fruits: how to combine citrus with grapefruit in your deodorant

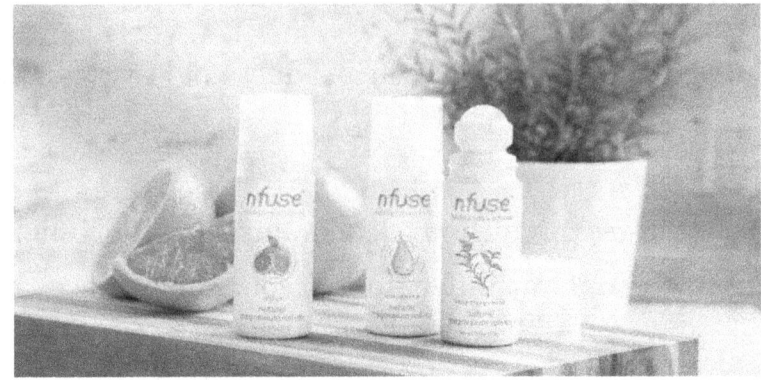

Liquid natural deodorant at home is the easiest to prepare. It consists almost entirely of vegetable oils, which are strictly metered and selected in such a way as not to leave greasy marks on clothes. To make a liquid deodorant at home with your own hands, you will need 5 milliliters of grape seed oil (as well, you might use sesame instead), 7-10 drops of tea tree oil, 5 drops of rosemary oil (you can substitute geranium oil or palmarosa), 15 drops of lavender oil, and bottle deodorant roller

Grape seed oil contributes to the rapid absorption and drying of funds, tea tree gives an excellent antiseptic, and various essential oils are added to bring a pleasant aroma to the composition. All components after adding to the bottle should be thoroughly shaken. If it is not possible to add all the listed oils, then you can use only the required - grape seed oil, tea tree and rosemary.

In the warm season, try not to use deodorant orange, lemon and grapefruit oil for making your own hands. They are very susceptible to the heat of the sun and if you go to sunbathe using this tool, you run the risk of severe burns.

Inflicting deodorant, it should be allowed to soak. This will happen within 5-7 minutes. You can store it for 3 weeks in a dry dark place. Such a deodorant, cooked with your own hands, does not leave marks on clothes and perfectly eliminates unpleasant odor. If you feel that the aroma has evaporated, you can safely add a few drops of a little heated essential oil to the composition.

It is believed it that the following citrus recipe for **homemade deodorant** originates in ancient Egypt, and it was used by verily famous Queen Cleopatra. Take the juice of your favorite citrus and mix it with a small amount of cinnamon. Pay attention that as a result of mixing you should get a mixture that has the consistency, like sour cream. As well, you might add in the following substance some rose oil that should be applied in a small amount. As a deodorant, such a combination which included rose oil it was first used in India. To make the effect better, before applying, mix rose oil with any base oil (olive, peach and so on): for one tablespoon of base oil, 6 drops of rose oil.

Citrus homemade deodorant will be perfect for everyone who loves the fresh aroma of oranges and lemons. For its manufacture will need 0.5 tablespoons of beeswax, 2 tablespoons of coconut oil, 2 tablespoons of baking soda, 1 tablespoon of corn starch, 10-15 drops of essential oil (you can use several flavors at once). Beeswax must be melted, then mix coconut oil with it. Soda and cornstarch should be poured into the resulting billet, mix thoroughly and add essential oils.

The mixture is placed in a tube and put to cool. Take your time using the deodorant you made. The finished mixture takes time to harden. As a rule, it is enough for this from several hours to one day. Apply a deodorant in a very thin layer, without pressure. If you did everything correctly, no trace of the product on the skin (and even more so on clothing) should remain.

Chapter 7 – Rose deodorants: when fragrance is the most important

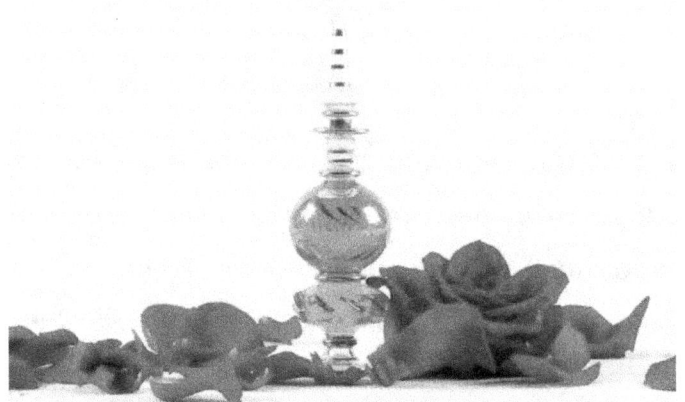

The deodorants with the rose components are usually based on the structure which you have already studied very well from the previous recipes. You might take the basis and add rose oil in such an amount which seems great for you. For example, let's look at the following recipe of **rose deodorant**.

Firstly, take 25 g of soda,15 g of corn starch, 30 g coconut oil, and rose oil. At the beginning, mix the right amount of soda with starch. Soda has long been considered the best way to combat the smell of sweat, because it creates an alkaline environment that destroys bacteria.

Starch absorbs moisture quickly, so the armpits will always be dry. Add coconut oil. It melts at 24 degrees, so when applied to the skin, the deodorant will melt slightly and slide well. You can also add a couple of drops of your favorite rose essential oil. Just remember that you will feel this smell all day, so choose a pleasant scent for yourself.

Place the resulting mass in a deodorant box, tamp well. This tool should be stored in the refrigerator. Self-made deodorant is harmless and does not violate the natural processes in the body. Of course, you need to get used to it, but the result will pleasantly surprise you. With proper use, such a deodorant is very economical, and you can check its effectiveness right now!

Liquid deodorant with alum also might contain the component of rose. It will bring you unforgettable fragrance. As well, it is hard while preparing. To make it, take 5 gr of aluminum alum, 40 gr of distilled water, Vitamin E, and 5 gr of Glycerin.

Additional ingredients are the following ones:
- *Shea butter - 5 gr.*
- *Rosemary hydrolat (deodorant itself) - 15 ml.*
- *Rose hydrolat (antibacterial properties) - 15 ml.*
- *Xanthan or guar (gelling agent) - 1 gr.*
- *Malavit (has healing and deodorizing qualities) - 30 cap.*
- *Aloe, liquid extract or aloe juice (moisturizes, relieves irritation) - 6 ml.*
- *Chlorophyllite alcohol (preservative) - 1 tsp.*
- *Essential oils are necessary, so jasmine and orange are well combined.*

To prepare it, do the following things:

1. Pour distilled water into a container, pour alum, put in a bath 40 degrees, stir until alum is dissolved.

2. Pour herbal distillate, xanthan or guar. At this stage, the water should be warm enough, but not boiling water, so that the hydrolates would not lose their properties. Mix well to dissolve the gel.

3. Add the remaining ingredients.

4. Beat with a blender or mixer, or just a fork.

5. Wash the bottle and roller of industrial deodorant, dry, spray it with alcohol to disinfect and pour deodorant.

Alum significantly reduces the secretion of sebaceous and sweat glands, is a strong antiperspirant, and has a deodorizing effect. Unlike aluminum, which is commonly used in industrial deodorants, which penetrates the blood and accumulates in the internal organs, forms plugs in the sweat glands, potassium alum does not penetrate into the cells and do not disrupt the work of the sweat glands.

Their action is based on high adsorption properties. Alum destroy bacterial cells, whose vital activity is the source of the smell. This deodorant absorbs quickly and pleasantly lubricates and moisturizes.